2-25-14

Living with Your Eye Operation

By THEODORE BERLAND

The Scientific Life

Your Children's Teeth
(WITH ALFRED E. SEYLER, D.D.S.)

X-ray—Vanguard of Modern Medicine

How to Keep Your Teeth After 30

Noise—The Third Pollution

The Fight for Quiet

Peptic Ulcer—the Quiet Epidemic

Living with Your Ulcer
(WITH MITCHELL A. SPELLBERG, M.D.)

Living with Your Bad Back
(WITH ROBERT G. ADDISON, M.D.)

Living with Your Bronchitis and Emphysema
(WITH GORDON L. SNIDER, M.D.)

LIVING WITH YOUR EYE OPERATION

Theodore Berland, A.M.
and
Richard Aloysius Perritt, M.D.,
F.A.A.O.O., F.I.C.S.

Clinical Professor of Ophthalmology, Cook County
Post-Graduate School of Medicine
Attending Ophthalmologist, Cook County Hospital
Executive Medical Director, Eye Rehabilitation and
Research Foundation
Senior attending Ophthalmologist,
Northwestern Memorial Hospitals
Assistant Professor of Ophthalmology,
Chicago Medical School
Attending Ophthalmologist, Henrotin Hospital

Illustrations by JUNE HILL PEDIGO

ST. MARTIN'S PRESS
New York

For Marvin and Frankie, whose vision is
beyond their sight.

T.B.

For my good patients, whose questions
deserve good answers.

R.A.P.

1. Clyde, Carmen, and the Cardinal

You wouldn't suspect it today, but for forty-four years, Clyde was blind. First of all, only one of his eyes is real. That he can see with it, is a miracle of modern surgery. Yet it is the kind of personal miracle which occurs every day in special operating rooms of the world's largest medical centers.

Clyde's close relatives remember that he was born with vision, and saw well as a baby. But at about two years of age, his sight began to fade. Doctors said an infection was the cause, and one eye was so badly destroyed it had to be removed. It was replaced with an artificial eye. Then they did what they could in those pre-antibiotic days to save the other. They half-succeeded. The eye remained, but all Clyde could see with it was light and dark; once in a while he could make out especially bright colors. Also, the infection seemed never to leave for good, recurring several times a year.

With no useful vision, Clyde was legally and practically blind and so he was reared and educated. After he grew up he was able to hold a job which required no vision; to marry, to raise a family, to work around the house and garden.

1

During these years, he had been happy and reverently thanked the Lord for the family's blessings every evening at dinner. Still, there were times when he longed to see. His children were growing quickly and (he was sure) beautifully. But he longed to see them, and to see his house, and the flowers he cherished. He longed to be able to play ball, as other fathers—sighted fathers—did with their sons. He longed to look in his wife's face and tell her how beautiful she was. He longed to see the many birds he heard in his garden, and to see the millions of things in his family's world which blindness kept him from sharing with them.

His chance came when he was forty-six. During a routine physical examination in his family doctor's office, he blurted out an answer that was so negative that it surprised even him. He was asked, "How have you been lately, Clyde?" He answered with a chuckle, "I'm OK, but I'd be a lot finer if I could get this eye out. It's always festering." The doctor sensed the tension behind the remark and made a little humming sound he always made when thinking. Finally, he said, "Well, let me see your eye, Clyde. Hmmmm. You know, it's been a long time since you lost that other eye. Lots of progress has been made in ophthalmology. Why don't I refer you to an eye doctor I know and let him examine you? You've got nothing to lose."

Clyde skeptically agreed. The ophthalmologist, however, wasn't too hopeful. He explained that he should be able to clear the infection once and for all, but that was only part of Clyde's problem. Over the years the recurring infection had done incredible damage to the cornea; this normally crystal-clear dome-shaped "front window" was, in Clyde's eye, scarred and opaque—the reason he could make out only light and dark, and not sharp images. The doctor offered Clyde little hope, other than to say that he advised against removing that eye at that time. "Some new technique may come along. You never know," the doctor advised.

By coincidence, the eye doctor was traveling through India

in the next few months and heard a lecture by a fellow American ophthalmologist (RAP), a Chicagoan, on microsurgical techniques for cutting away diseased corneas and replacing them with new corneas. Since Clyde and his eye doctor lived in Milwaukee, he called upon his return and set up an appointment for Clyde in Chicago with this expert.

In Chicago, Clyde's examination included a careful analysis of the infection (it was caused by the dread germ staphylococcus) and the wreckage it had wrought on the cornea. The Chicago surgeon told Clyde he felt he could not only stop the infection, but repair the cornea. But there were no guarantees. It would be a long process, accompanied by discomfort, pain, inconvenience, and expense. But if everything worked out, Clyde should actually be able to see in a few months.

Clyde was excited. He might be able to see! Still, it *could* fail. It was perhaps the most difficult decision Clyde ever had to make. He thought about it as he walked with his stick on busy streets, and on the train ride home, and he discussed what the doctor had said with his family. The next morning, he called Chicago and told the doctor he was prepared to go through with it.

The treatment took longer than the Chicago surgeon had estimated. The staph germ was so tough that four months of treatment with antibiotics, other medicines, and other techniques were required. Finally, the eye was clear of infection; then the cornea's heavy scarring was even more apparent. Equally apparent was the fact that for Clyde to see again, he would need a new cornea. He worried that one would be available to be placed in his eye.

The Chicago doctor's office called eye banks around the country, looking for a "fresh eye" from a cadaver. While it sounds grisly, it is in fact a beautiful gift. By willing his eyes, a person can give to the living after his or her death. The cornea—like the nails, hair, and other parts of the body —does not die instantly when the heart stops. It continues to live and thus can continue to give sight to another person.

One day, the New York Eye Bank called and said it had the eye of a man who had just been killed in an auto accident. Clyde was immediately notified and told to come to Chicago. At the same time, the operating-room supervisor of a Chicago hospital was notified that the eye was coming and that surgery would be performed the next day. Within two hours after the accident victim's death in New York, the complete eye was on its way to LaGuardia Airport, packed in a special container containing ice to keep it cool. Eastern Airlines flew the eye (at no cost) to O'Hare International Airport, where a Red Cross courier picked it up and whisked it to the downtown Chicago hospital. The next day, the cornea of the still-living eye of a dead New Yorker was transplanted to the long-blind eye of the living Milwaukeean.

What Clyde saw and felt after the operation is best told by himself, in a letter he wrote later to the Chicago surgeon. He tells of a suspense like that in a movie, as the bandages were removed. He told of his feelings: "I could see everyone around my bed and gave a short cry of joy with many strained and sobbing exclamations."

After several more weeks in the hospital, his wife took him home. He made the trip with his eye bandaged for protection. At home his wife removed the bandage for the last time. He could see! In fact, the light was so brilliant it hurt his eye at first. "It took about an hour before I was able to keep my eye open. I was in the kitchen at the time and it was wonderful to see the marble design on the floor. I looked at the cabinets—and never knew wood could be so pretty! By this time the tears were flowing and with our family all together it seemed like Christmas Eve to me."

With his wife's help, he walked through the house, for the first time seeing the colors of walls, pictures, and furniture. "I told my wife I hated to go to bed that night for fear that I would wake and find that it was a dream," he wrote. But he could see again when he awakened the next morning and he felt brave enough to go down and make breakfast for the two of them. "I was amazed at the bright yellow of the egg yolks," he exclaimed.

"It was sure good to put the dishes on the table without having to feel just where to put everything. My wife came to the kitchen and we sat down to a very happy breakfast together. Being in the habit (as she always was) of taking care of me by pouring my coffee or milk, even buttering my bread, she was ready to do the same thing this morning, but I told her that from now on I was going to try and do things for her the way she did them for me. Even when I poured milk in my glass she was ready to stop me. However, when I filled it to the proper level, she just smiled."

In the afternoon, his daughter took him into the garden. "I love flowers, especially roses," he explained. "I liked to feel the smooth petals, but my wife used to tell me that I killed the blossoms that way. Now I was able to see them! Their colors were brilliant and breathtaking. It seemed as though they waited to bloom until I came home. They were beautiful."

Every subsequent day was filled with wonderful new sights. He discovered sunshine, and grass and lawn furniture. He also discovered new activities. Ever since he had been a schoolboy, he had wanted to play ball. One Sunday after his operation "the men were out in the yard tossing a football around when my son-in-law called to me from a distance of about sixty feet. He said, 'Can you catch, Dad?' I looked toward him when he threw the ball lightly to me and to his surprise I reached out and caught the ball. They really had someone standing in back of me at the time figuring that I would miss anyway. You can imagine the surprise on their faces when I caught it. Everyone let out a yell."

Not long after he had been home, he attended a picnic at the local Home for the Blind. Although he didn't live there, he had worked on the entertainment committee for a number of years. He very much wanted to go to the picnic and (literally) see his old friends. Of course, word of his operation and its success had preceded him, so that when he arrived, he was swamped; his blind friends wanted to touch him and to shake his hand. "I felt as though I were the President of the United States," he recalled. "But I couldn't see them at first. The tears in my eye were swelled up so. Then I could see that even the eight or so seeing-eye dogs around were looking at me."

A disturbing aspect of Clyde's new vision was riding in an automobile. The panorama moved by so fast that it made him feel almost dizzy. After all, he was not used to seeing still things, let alone trees and cars which whisked by. But since these early days, he understands motion and even drives a car. He has also given up the routine use of braille and has learned to read and write by sight. In fact, he finished his first letter to his doctor by stating that it was most amazing that "I am able at this time, without the aid of glasses, to glance over the top of this typewriter and actually read what I write."

Personal miracles such as that experienced by Clyde have also come to the famous. Another man whom surgery helped to see again was the Welterweight and Middleweight Champion of the World, Carmen Basilio. He was temporarily blinded because of the terrible punishment his eyes had received from injuries during years of boxing; his blindness was precipitated by the gloves of "Sugar" Ray Robinson during a bout in Chicago. The morning after the fight, Basilio's darkened eyelids were swollen shut and caked with blood. His handlers had lanced the puffed lids with a razor to let blood out in order to relieve the swelling, but that had done little good.

The Champ, as his handlers called him, was rushed to Wesley Hospital for emergency treatment. First, the eye surgeon administered medicine to reduce as much as possible the swelling and inflammation of the eyelids. Then Basilio was taken to the operating rooms where large, stringy blood clots, which had formed behind his eyeballs, were removed.

Then the lids were carefully trimmed to remove the scars of this and past fights, and were sewn together again with the delicate and precise techniques of plastic surgery. When Basilio's bandages were removed, he saw again; he recovered so fully that he went on and fought many more matches.

Another uncommon man whom eye operations (also by RAP) helped to see, this one dedicated to peace, was Thomas Cardinal Tien, S.V.D., Archbishop of Peking, who came to America in 1951 after refusing the office of "Pope of China" cynically proffered by the Communist regime. The fifty-nine-year-old prelate was essentially blind; he could just distinguish light and darkness; he could not even perceive shadows. His blindness was the result of an incredible assortment of eye troubles: in each eye a segment of the cataract was bound by scar tissue to the liquid inside the eye; also, the internal pressure of the eyeball was dangerously high, producing glaucoma; and, finally, the inside of the eye contained clots of blood and thick scar tissue.

Two years after his arrival in New York, Cardinal Tien was taken to Chicago. The chancery office there made arrangements for him to be examined and, if necessary, operated on. He was taken to Wesley Hospital, where he was examined, and placed on a special diet to prepare his body for the operations. His years of deprivation in China had had their effect: he was emaciated from hunger, and also had a kidney infection. After ten days of food and intravenous fluids and treatment of his infection he was ready for surgery.

The area to be opened in his right eye was less than that of a dime: looking through a special microscope focused on the clear part of the left eye, the surgeon's steady hands delicately manipulated instruments to remove the cloudy remnant of the cataract, as well as scar tissue and all traces of infection and bleeding. A month later, at Columbus Hospital, the same was done for the other eye. Weeks later, the bandages were removed in the surgeon's office, and both eyes were examined. The surgeon found the Columbus (or Catholic) eye better than the Wesley (Methodist) eye. Tests showed that seventy percent of his vision was restored. With glasses to further aid his eyes, Cardinal Tien returned to Taiwan to continue his work for seventeen more years before he died.

Clyde, Carmen and the Chinese cardinal are real people, each of whom was once blind, and whose sight was restored by surgery. They are among the million or so in the world each year whose eyes are operated on to regain their vision or to see better. As a reader of this book, you or your relative or friend, will soon be among the legions of happy people who are made to see again with surgery.

There are no operations like eye operations. The ophthalmologist (eye surgeon) works on a ball-shaped organ about an inch in diameter. In a visually oriented society, it is perhaps the most important organ of perception, continually feeding thousands of bits of information to the brain, giving us the ability to gauge distances, appreciate the beauty of colors, perceive motion without experiencing it, and instantly recognize the moods and feelings of our loved ones—among its other blessings. The ophthalmologist must himself have excellent vision; he operates with the aid of a microscope and uses sutures that are thinner than human hair. His hand must be steady; his nerves steellike.

Because it is so important, and so complex, and because so many things can go wrong with it, the eye has been the concern of doctors since the dawn of medicine. In ancient Egypt, each eye of the pharaoh had its own keeper. The mysteries of the eye so fascinated these early people, that they ascribed it as the symbol of Horus, the falcon-god. Horus, according to mythology, was bent on avenging the death of his father, Osiris, who had been god-king of the earth. Horus fought with the murderer, Set, but in the fight Horus's eye was ripped from its socket (or *orbit*) and torn into six fragments. Thoth, the ibis-god, reassembled the eye, miraculously healed it and replaced it. As a result, the sign of Horus is also used as a symbol of healing.

In the ninth century B.C. embalmers removed the eyes of dead important Egyptians, poured wax or plaster into the orbits and inserted precious stones. In the fifth century B.C., Roman priests who practiced surgery replaced diseased eyes with artificial ones. These were much cruder than the glass eyes made in Venice after 1579.

The first corneal transplant was performed in 1835 by a British army surgeon; it was on a pet gazelle. Seventy years later the first human corneal transplant was performed by Dr. Eduard Zirm in Austria. The first successful operation for glaucoma (*iridectomy*) was performed in Germany by Albrecht von Graefe in about 1850.

It was the invention of the operating microscope (first used in surgery by RAP in 1946), and the availability of extremely fine sutures and needles, which opened the way to the tremendous proliferation of eye operations occurring in our lifetime. Within a generation, surgery of the eye changed from a rare oddity to a much-practiced specialty. (In fact, eye surgeons were the first to be certified as specialists.) Today, around the United States more than half a million eye operations are performed every year.* More operations are performed on the eye than on peptic ulcers, hemorrhoids, or gallstones; the eye is more frequently operated on than are the nose, ear, breast, brain, heart, appendix, prostate, or bone joints. Eye operations are among the fifty most frequently performed kinds of surgery in hospitals** and a leading cause of hospitalization.***

*Surgery in Short-Stay Hospitals: United States, 1968. *Monthly Vital Statistics Report*, 21: 5-6, Supplement 2 (9 June) 1972.
**The Fifty Most Frequent Operations, 1964, *The Record*, Vol. 3, No. 9 (10 December) 1965.
***The Leading Causes of Admission, PAS Hospitals, 1964, *The Record*, Vol. 3, No. 11 (31 January) 1966.

We'll give you, your family, and friends a few more statistics, so that you can all understand how typical is the experience.

In terms of age, eye operations are most frequently performed on children and old people. According to one government report,* "Operations associated with the orbit, eyeball, and ocular muscles ranked second for those under fifteen years of age or at four times the rate of older groups." But two-thirds of cataract operations (*extraction of lens*) are performed on adults sixty-five years of age or older.

Eye surgery can't cure all eye ills, nor return vision to all the blind. But it is the hope of many, such as you. The data from the National Center for Health Statistics indicate that 1,342,000 Americans have no useful vision; if they have eyesight, it is so poor that they cannot read ordinary newspaper print with glasses. They mainly suffer from cataract, glaucoma, and retina diseases. ** According to the U.S. Welfare Administration, 95,000 Americans are on the public assistance rolls for aid to the blind.

Perhaps because we rely so on our eyes (it is said that ninety percent of the information which forms the basis of our knowledge and information comes visually), we all dread blindness. A Gallup survey conducted in cooperation with Research to Prevent Blindness, Inc., in 1965 found that "next to cancer, the disease or ailment which is most feared by the American people is blindness." It is more dreaded than heart disease, arthritis, polio, loss of a limb, tuberculosis, or deafness, the survey found.

The purpose of this book is not to frighten you further, nor to unduly alarm you (while we use "you," we will, in this book, mean the patient, or a relative, or a friend). Our

---

Surgical Operations in Short-Stay Hospitals (Series 13, No. 7). Rockville, Md.: National Center for Health Statistics. 1971.
**Selected Impairments* (Series 10, No. 48). Washington: National Center for Health Statistics, 1968.

objective is to give you all of the background and facts you need to understand your eye condition; how your problem developed; and, why your doctor recommends the operation he does.

You have to be able to properly assess, with your doctor's help, of course, your situation. You are not suffering from anything as slight as a cold. Your eye problem won't disappear by itself. But it no doubt is amenable to surgical treatment.

We will not go into great detail here about such subjects as eyeglasses and contact lenses, except as they are involved in postsurgical treatment. Nor will we spend much time on other general eye problems, such as color blindness or presbyopia. Instead, the focus of this book is on conditions treated by surgery. After surgery, you will have to learn to live with your eye condition. We hope this book can help make that possible and less painful.

Because your vision is at stake, you must place yourself in the hands of a competent surgeon. If you follow his advice and take care of yourself after the operation as he directs, you can regain your vision and live what will be an essentially normal life. But if you do not, you are gambling with your eyesight.

Since your way of life, and indeed your life itself, are in your hands, we think you will be properly and powerfully motivated to accept your doctor's plan of treatment and personal care. It will not all be easy or convenient, but it will all be essential.

We intend in this book to give you all of the background and facts you need to understand your eyes and their disorder and how it developed.

Besides telling you the pertinent anatomy and physiology of your eyes, this book will also tell you in detail the most likely operation you can expect for your condition.

We assume that the reader of this book is an adult, and so the information that follows is intended to be conveyed from one adult to another. There is no attempt here to sugar-coat and no attempt to substitute cute nicknames for real names, although, to help your understanding, we will also use popular, commonly used terms for parts of the eye, for diseases, or for conditions.

As you read this book, remember that it is a tool you should use with good judgment. No book can replace the skills and services of your personal physician. His diagnosis and prescribed plan of treatment in all cases must supersede anything said here. If there is any controversy or contradiction between what is printed here and what he says, take his word against ours.

On the other hand, the information included here should help spare you the need to ask your doctor to give you a short medical education in the pathogenesis, diagnosis, and treatment of various eye disorders. It should also inform you of the facts you want or need, but are too rushed or ashamed to ask of him. We also hope that this book saves your doctor some time and explanation.

In other words, this book is designed to help you see and to help you live with your eye condition. If it does that, it will have achieved its purpose and its authors' intention.

If you've come this far, to the point where you realize you need an eye operation, then the chance is good that you already have an eye surgeon. If not, you may wonder how to find one. Here is a quick guide.

The best way to find a surgeon is the way you would find any doctor: by referral or recommendation. You may know somebody who has been treated by a doctor and has been happy with him and the results. Or you may be referred by your minister, priest, or rabbi, or a social agency—especially if you are new in town. Or, your family physician may refer you.

For eye surgery you need an ophthalmologist. That is the

technical name for an eye surgeon, an M.D. who specializes in the eye. There are about 5,000 in the United States.

There are other kinds of health professionals who deal with the eye, so don't become confused. An *optometrist* (O.D.) examines your eyes for glasses or contact lenses, but uses no drugs and performs no surgery (he may also grind lenses and sell glasses); an *optician* grinds lenses and sells glasses, but does no examination, prescribes no drugs, and does no surgery. *Oculist* is an old term for M.D.s who specialized in eyes but usually did no surgery.

Once you have the name of an ophthalmologist, check his credentials. Call your local medical society and ask, or go to the public library or a hospital library and look him up in *Directory of Medical Specialists*. You can also check with the American Medical Association, 535 North Dearborn Street, Chicago, Illinois 60610. If he is an osteopathic eye surgeon (he'll have the initials D.O. after his name, instead of M.D.), you can check with the American Osteopathic Association, 212 East Ohio Street, Chicago, Illinois 60611.

The most important credential is certification by the American Board of Ophthalmology. This assures you of his competence as a surgeon who specializes in the eye. A doctor becomes certified only after a rigorous set of examinations; today a surgeon doesn't even qualify to take the examination until he has finished residency training, which means about four years of specialized education in a hospital after he has graduated from medical school and finished his internship.

Another important credential is membership in the American College of Surgeons (often indicated by the initials F.A.C.S., for "Fellow, American College of Surgeons") or the American College of Osteopathic Surgeons. Many eye surgeons are also Fellows of the International College of Surgeons, or F.I.C.S.

Even more important is membership in the American Academy of Ophthalmology and Otolaryngology (indicated by the initials, F.A.A.O.O.). This means that the eye surgeon is not only educated and has proved his competence, but also keeps up-to-date on new developments and changes in the specialty by a program of continuing education.

If the doctor recommended to you has the proper credentials, you are pretty well assured of his competence. But there are still a few cautions to observe. Be wary of the doctor who wants to rush you to the operating room. An ethical doctor will:

> —Answer your questions, in as much detail as you need.
> —Explain the alternatives to surgery.
> —Tell you of the possible benefits and complications of the operation.
> —Be willing to discuss fees.
> —Be willing to have you consult another eye surgeon.

Don't be a doctor-shopper and call on every eye surgeon you can find for his opinion of your case. But it is quite all right to seek out another competent eye surgeon and let him examine you and see if he recommends an operation and, if so, what kind. The eye surgeon should be willing to refer you to one of his colleagues; or, if you would rather, get the name of another through your family physician, the medical society, or one of the reference books. You should know that it is ethically improper for a doctor to refuse you this right of consultation with another specialist. Nor should you make a quest of searching for an eye doctor who tells you what you want to hear, no matter how long it takes. While you don't want to be rushed into surgery, your disease is not likely to get any better without treatment.

Don't let the cautions we have proposed scare you. Once you have agreed to the operation, be positive in your outlook. Be assured that you have made the right decision, that the operation will restore your vision and that you will see better than you have for a long time.

2. Understanding Your Eyes

Your eyes are your windows to the world. Physically they are two liquid-containing globes set in watery sockets in your skull. Poetically they are as Tennyson wrote in *Idylls of the King*, "wholesome stars of love." Practically, they are your sensory organs of vision. In modern mechanistic terms, they are light-sensors linked to your central data handler, your brain, in the system known as *vision* or *sense of sight*. Eyes that function normally and healthily, automatically and very efficiently feed a constant stream of information to the brain.

Your eyes are the product of perhaps half a billion years of evolution. Forms of life on earth have sensed light from almost the first brilliant moment of creation. Green plants require light to live; they will bend, twist and otherwise contort themselves into strange shapes in order to best expose themselves to light. Even the lowly one-celled amoeba is sensitive to light. The earthworm, which also has no eyes, has skin which is sensitive to light so it can burrow into the damp earth as the sun rises to dry the air. If you've ever gathered night crawlers to fish with, you know that they scramble for cover when the beam of your flashlight shines on them.

Creatures' eyes have an amazing variety of locations, sizes, and shapes to best serve in hunting or escaping a hunter. Thus hawks and eagles have extremely keen, long-range sight; owls have wonderful night vision; and the rabbit's eyes are so located that it can see any of these hunters attacking from behind.

The variety of eyes seems endless. Scallops have rows of eyes just inside their shells, while the eyes of the conch are on the ends of its tentacles. Crabs have eyes like periscopes and spiders have clusters of eyes. The horsefly's eyes cover most of its head; each eye has 7,000 facets. The bottom-dwelling flounder has both eyes on the same, upward-facing side, so it can look up through the water. Fish and snakes can't blink their eyes; lizards blink their eyes by raising their lower lids (we drop our upper lid).

Human eyes are unique in that they both face forward, move, provide three-dimensional vision, see colors, rapidly shift focus as distances change, adapt to light levels, and can perceive motion.

That the eye is usually compared with a camera is no coincidence; the camera, of course, was designed long after the human eye. For about two thousand years scientists thought of and experimented with ways to form direct images. Since the first man saw his world, images have been drawn, etched, painted, carved and formed with hands, and with instruments manipulated by hands.

The trick was to find a way to have the light waves themselves form the images. It was a canny German Jesuit, Christopher Scheiner, who in 1625 proved that the eye forms images directly from light. He took the eye of a newly slaughtered animal and scraped away the opaque white coating on the back so that all that was left was a translucent membrane. Then he held the eye in front of his own and pointed it at an object, perhaps a crucifix. On that membrane was an inverted image of the crucifix! He thought it truly a miracle.

Actually, Father Scheiner was merely confirming what

Leonardo da Vinci had proposed about a century before. To demonstrate his theory of how the eye sees, he used two rooms, one well-lighted, one dark. He made a tiny hole in the wall between the rooms; standing in the dark room, he held a piece of paper close to the small light hole. When he adjusted the paper to the proper distance from the hole, inverted images were formed of objects in the lighted room. Leonardo didn't invent the *camera obscura* (it had been used since antiquity); but he was the first to understand how it works and its relation to the eye.

Taken from the Latin words for dark room, the camera obscura is just that: a darkened room in which you can see images of the sunlit world without.

The seventeenth century was an important time for optics. Observations of how animal and human eyes work led to deeper investigations of optics, the invention of the telescope by a Dutch lens grinder named Lippershey, its refinement by Galileo, and the formulations of the laws of refraction by Snell and Descartes, Grimaldi, Hooke, Newton, Huygens and Fresnel.

A major application of optics over a century later was the invention of photography in 1839 by Louis Daguerre and William Fox Talbot. They made it possible for light images to be recorded and kept permanently.

But the human eye forms and transmits images; it doesn't record them. The development of the television camera in the 1920s came a little closer. Mechanically and electronically, it captures images and transmits them.

The analogy of TV camera to eye is not perfect—nor will it ever be between the human eye and a mechanical device—but it may help you to understand the anatomy of your eye and how each part works. Once you understand these basic principles and facts, you will have a better understanding of your eye problem, the operation you need, and the reason you need it.

In order that you may completely understand the eye, we'll

first give you a general description of how it works and what the parts of the eye do to make it work. Then we'll go into a more detailed description.

Leonardo was quite right. The eye essentially is a dark chamber with a small opening for letting light in. There is a small, dark circle at the center of the eye which changes size. Through this circle—the *pupil* of the eye—you are looking into the eye. You see only blackness because the inside of the eye, like Leonardo's chamber, is dark.

This biological dark chamber is a nearly perfect globe. It has a bulge at the front which you can see when you look at an eye in profile. This bulge contains the light-gathering apparatus of the eye. The "skin" of the entire eyeball is opaque to light except at this bulge, where it is normally a beautifully clear and round window called the *cornea*. The cornea gathers light rays and directs them to the lens just behind. Because the intensity of light sources outside varies from sunlight to moonlight, the eye (like the TV camera) has a device for keeping fairly constant the amount of light which enters the dark chamber. This is the *iris*, a name shared by eye and camera, and located between the light focusing elements. The lens—like the lens of a TV camera—focuses the light rays to form an image at the back of the eye. As in a TV camera, the image is inverted and backward.

The inside lining of the eye on which the image is focused is called the *retina* (a camera has been named after it!). The retina, like the signal plate of a TV camera, is actually a mosaic made of many thousands of light-sensitive elements; these convert the image to impulses which are transmitted to another location. In the case of the TV camera, these are electronic impulses that are then broadcast so that receivers can reconstitute them as images of what the TV camera sees. In the case of the retina, these are nerve impulses which are conducted to the brain, where the image is reconstituted and, as we say, perceived. In both cases, there are mechanisms

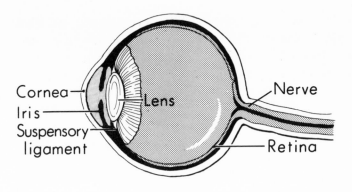

Cornea
Iris
Suspensory
ligament
Lens
Nerve
Retina

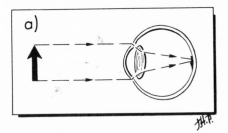

a)

FIG. 1. Anatomy and Function. The normal eye seen here in cross section acts like a television camera to form continuously changing images of the world. The cornea gathers light for the lens, which focuses it on the retina at the rear. The focusing power of the lens is adjusted by the suspensory ligament. In front of the lens is the iris, which opens and closes to keep constant the amount of light entering the eye. The inverted image is converted by the retina to nervous impulses; these are transmitted by the optic nerve to the brain.

built in to right and to reverse the upside-down, backwards image formed inside the dark chamber.

The nerve impulses are integrated in the brain and compared there with other information which that marvelous biological data center receives from your other senses—especially hearing, touch, and balance. Usually, all of the information from these senses makes sense; that is, agrees. But there are instances when the data disagree. One instance is dizziness, when your eyes tell you they are level with the horizon, but your inner ear (where balance is sensed) says you are tilted. Or when your eyes say an object is two-and-a-half feet in front of your nose but that object is not there when you go to grasp it. Or when you hear a siren, as you drive your car, but cannot see the direction from which the fire engine is racing at you through the streets.

Human eyes can move, and they can move in rather wide sweeps, sideways and up-and-down. Usually, eyes are coordinated so that they are both focused on the same object, whether it is as close as the tip of your nose or as far away as the moon. The fact that your eyes are on either side of your nose, separated by two and one half inches or so, means that each eye sees the same object, but sees it slightly differently. When information from these slightly different images—one from the right and one from the left—are put together in the brain, the result of this *binocular vision* is that you see the world in 3-D; the world, as you perceive it by light, is not a flat picture like a cartoon or a photograph, but is three-dimensional, with near objects standing out sharply from the background of more distant objects, and they less sharply from the more general and distant background behind them. In effect, you see around objects—more around close objects and less around distant objects. This gives you depth perception. Coupled with movement, this helps you to judge distances and speed. You note this when you look up at the sky and see several layers of clouds: the lower ones move faster and look rounder than the high, slow-moving clouds.

Your eyes are also served by cleverly designed accessories. The most apparent are the eyelids, which cover and protect the eyes as we sleep. The lids also automatically blink when wind threatens to dry the eyes, or when dust blows to irritate them. Blinking your eyelids, like running the wipers over your automobile's windshield, sweeps dirt away.

In the edges of the eyelids are tiny glands which secrete

oil to prevent the edges of the upper and lower lids from sticking together during your sleep. The oil also serves as a barrier to keep the normal level of tears from spilling over the edge. Also growing out of these edges, of course, are the *lashes* which, when they blink every ten seconds or so, sweep dust and lint out of the air that is immediately in front of your eyes. Eyebrows are there to keep the dirty sweat of your brow from running into your eyes.

The tears are the ''windshield washers'' of your eyes. They also lubricate your eyes so the lids can glide smoothly over them. Tears are produced by a small gland hidden behind the upper lid at the outer corner of the eye. The tears, which are salty and slightly antiseptic, flow from this gland through ducts under the lids and cross the cornea to keep it moist and clean. The tears collect at the inner corner of the eye, then drain through a duct into the nose. Normally, the flow and drainage of tears is in perfect balance so that the front of the eye is moist. But with disease or emotion, tears may flood up and spill over (callous as it sounds, that is what happens in crying), or diminish, producing dry eyes. The entire tear works system of the eye is called the *lacrimal apparatus*.

Finally, the eye is well protected because it is literally located in a hole in your skull, the eyesocket, or *orbit*. This means that all but direct blows to the eye are fended off by bone.

Now that you have a general idea of how the eye works, and the parts that make it work, let's get down to smaller details. We'll do this by starting with the outside of the eye and moving inward; and, from the cornea, or front of the eye, to the retina, or back of the eye.

The eyeball (also called the *globe*) has a three-layered ''skin.'' (These layers are also called the *coats* or *tunics*.) The outermost coat is tough and fibrous. Over most of the eyeball it is the *sclera*, colored white to reflect light, and opaque to prevent other outside light from diffusing into the dark *vitreous chamber*, which serves as the camera obscura of the eye. This same coat becomes miraculously transparent and bulges in a convex shape (in health) at the front of the eye to form the cornea. Surrounding the cornea and folding back to cover the inside of the lids is a protective mucous membrane, the conjunctiva, better known when it is irritated and red in the condition known as *conjunctivitis*.

The middle coat of the eye is even more complicated. At the back of the eye, it is essentially a continuous layer. Called the *choroid*, it spans five-sixths of the area of the eyeball to serve its dual function of helping keep light out, and providing blood vessels to nourish the innermost layer, the retina (see below).

At the front of the eye, the middle coat is not so simple: it separates into other structures with very specialized functions. One of these is the *iris*, a thin and lacy but muscular lifesaver-shaped membrane. The iris is what gives you the color of your eyes. When you were born, your iris had only two layers (that is why all babies have blue eyes). In brown eyes, the deeper, third layer (dark, like the choroid) forms a few weeks or months after birth, darkening the total color of the iris.

The iris is fascinating in many ways. As we explained earlier, its main purpose is to regulate the amount of light which passes through the lens. This is important, since too much light will cause glare and a distortion of the image; and, too little light will produce an indistinct image. The hole or opening which the iris shapes, the *pupil*, varies in size from the diameter of a pinhead to that of a pencil. The size of the pupil is regulated by an automatic control system after which automatic cameras are patterned. If the intensity of light which reaches the back of the eye is too great, then "too-strong" signals are sent over nerves to a deep part of the center of the brain, which sends back a motor signal to the iris to make the pupil smaller and cut down the light. If the light that enters the eye is too weak, the brain tells the iris to open up the pupil.

The iris opens and closes usually without your being aware of it, as when you go indoors and then out again. But if you are on the beach or a boat in the tropics, with the sun bright above you and also reflected from the water below, your iris will contract so tightly you may feel pain; also, your eyelids will automatically start to close in a squint to help keep light out.

There are other conditions which affect the size of the pupil. One is drugs, such as the drops which the doctor may place in your eye to relax the iris muscles so that the pupil dilates, or opens wide. Also, certain drugs which are injected or swallowed can act to dilate the pupils; narcotics have this effect, for instance. To give their eyes black brilliance, Italian Renaissance ladies took belladonna to dilate their pupils.

The pupil is also affected by the closeness of the object you are looking at: it closes down a bit to sharpen the image when you are reading, modelmaking, sewing, or doing other close work.

Emotions provoke the brain to open the iris. Thus, researchers at Southampton University in England explain, this is one reason watchmakers and others who do close work so detest noise, because it will provoke the pupils to widen, and ruin the fine focus their eyes have established. Also, Dr. Eckhard H. Hess of the University of Chicago found that men's pupils widen at the sight of a Playmate of the Month, while the pupils of women widen at the sight of a male pinup or a picture of a baby. Recently it was "discovered" that Chinese merchants have used this phenomenon for centuries. They know they can get a handsome price for jade when the customer's eyes widen, indicating he wants *that* item.

At the moment of death, the iris (like other muscles) relaxes, and the pupils widen for the last time.

The iris covers the *crystalline lens*, an equally remarkable part of the eye. While the cornea has some lenslike qualities of gathering light and focusing them, it is the lens which finally forms the image that is projected onto the retina at the back of the eye. Unlike the solid glass or plastic lens of a camera or telescope, the lens of the eye is made of more than two thousand fine layers that lie one on top of the other like the layers of a Bermuda onion. Each layer is made of fibers in a fingerprintlike pattern. It is because these layers and fibers get in the way that light from very weak sources, such as a star or a distant candle, seems to have tiny rays.

Unlike a camera lens, the lens of the eye is flexible. It has to be. The lens of a TV camera is moved back or forth to focus an image on the electronic charge plate at the back. There is a constant ratio that must be maintained of the distance of the lens to the subject in front, and to the plate in the back. Shellfish accomplish this by changing the shape of their eyeballs. Some fishes move their entire eyeball forward or backward to focus on objects. Birds change the shape of their cornea.

Human eyes, however, focus by changing the shape of the lens. Called *accommodation*, it is accomplished by a radiating muscular structure called the *ciliary body*. Focus is usually automatic, but can be overridden by conscious effort, such as when you stare out blankly into open space in deep meditation. As untiring as the heart muscle or the diaphragm involved in breathing, the ciliary body pulls on the *suspensory ligament* at the edge of the lens when you look into the distance. This flattens the lens. But when you are looking at something close, as at this book, those radiating muscle fibers relax and the circular ligament acts to contract the lens so that it is thick and more convex and better for focusing on close objects.

Dramatic as the focusing is in seeing, the physical dimensions which produce this are amazingly small: the lens doesn't change thickness by more than one-fiftieth of an inch!

We'll talk about lens troubles which need surgery in later chapters. But you should realize that the automatic, self-focusing system of the eye is not always perfect. For one thing, the suppleness of the lens slowly diminishes as a person ages. This means that it does not change focus so quickly when you read a newspaper, then look up at the television screen, and then look back at your paper. Usually this reduction in the ability of the lens to accommodate is noticed when a person is between forty and forty-five years of age. This is called *presbyopia*.

For another thing, the lens does not always focus a perfect picture, even in childhood. This means that another lens which is outside the eye has to supplement the cornea-lens focusing system. This is when glasses or contact lenses are needed. When the image falls short of the retina, this is near-sightedness or *myopia*; when the image is behind the retina, this is farsightedness or *hyperopia*. When the cornea is not perfectly round but has another bulge in it, *astigmatism* is the result; here the image is distorted so that parts are more in focus in the vertical plane than in the horizontal, or vice versa—much like those funny mirrors at the carnival or amusement park.

The *retina*, as we've said, is the inner lining or innermost coat of the eyeball. The retina looks like a pink net (its name means "net" in Latin). It receives a great deal of nutrition in the way of blood supply from the coat behind, the choroid; it receives its image of light from the cornea and lens in front. The retina is like the charge plate of a TV camera in that it is a mosaic of microscopic elements which are sensitive to light; they absorb the energy of light and convert it to electrical energy. The electrical energy is then transmitted to form an image elsewhere.

These sensitive elements, or photoreceptors, are of two kinds: *rods* and *cones*. The cones are spread all across the retina but are packed together most closely, as in a box of incense cones, toward the rear of the eye. This dense area of photoreceptors opposite the lens is called the *macula* and is where you see the best details in bright light. In technical terms, this is where the eye has the greatest visual acuity. Most of the eye's seven million cones are located here. This also is where the eye best perceives color. A tiny depression in the macula, the *fovea*, which is not exactly opposite the center of the lens, is the most sensitive area of the retina. One reason for the macula's acuity is that each cone is connected to a nerve fiber.

The eye's 130 million rods are distributed over the rest of the retina, mixed with cones and sharing nerve fibers. The rods are best at perceiving dim images, such as those of the night, and motion. But they do not perceive color, which is one reason everything is moody and dramatic in moonlight or streetlight. You see best in near-darkness by moving your eyes so that the light falls on rods, not the cones at the fovea.

The nerve fibers connected to the photoreceptors of the retina join larger and larger nerve fibers until they make up the rather thick optic nerve which stems out from the back of the eyeball around the artery and vein which supply and drain blood from the retina.

The spot at which the optic nerve leaves the eye is called the *optic disk*. Because there are no photoreceptors right there, this part of the retina does not sense light; that is why it is called the *blind spot*. Away from the eyeball, the optic nerve is like a TV cable meandering through the skull and into the brain.

Something interesting happens in this transmission system that doesn't happen in TV. The nerves from photoreceptors on the right sides of *both* eyes, cross over to the left side of the brain, and those from the left halves of both eyes to the right side of the brain. The occipital cortex, the surface of the brain way at the back of your head, is where the image is perceived.

We've given you the general concept of how the eye sees, as well as a detailed description of the parts that make it see. There is one more concept which is necessary for you to understand: once light is captured by the cornea, it travels through fluids until it is displayed as an image on the retina. The first fluid which that light passes through is the *aqueous humor*, a salty, watery substance which fills that space between the cornea and the lens, known as the *anterior chamber*. Aqueous humor is produced by the ciliary body. Like a river, and like the tears outside the eye, aqueous humor is constantly flowing: from the ciliary body through the opening in the iris, under the cornea, and is drained off by a tiny duct called *Schlemm's canal* found underneath the sclera adjacent to the cornea.

The much larger and dark camera-obscura chamber of the eye is filled with a jellylike substance known as the *vitreous humor*. Derived from the plasma of blood flowing through the choroid, it is ninety-nine percent water and one percent solids. It helps keep the eyeball round and firm as well as serving as the medium through which light is projected from the lens. It is not always perfect; in some people little bits of solids called *floaters* do just that—float around and appear like dust or spots. It is because light is somewhat bent as it travels through this jellylike medium that the fovea is not exactly opposite the center of the lens, as it would be in a camera filled with air.

We have not spent much attention here on the wonderful muscles of the eyes which move them right and left, up and down, and round and round. We'll explain them in detail in the next chapter, when we explain surgery for muscle imbalance.

3. Muscle Operations

If you need an eye muscle operation, it is because something is wrong with the complex system which usually keeps both eyes perfectly fixed on what you want to see. We intentionally did not describe these muscles before; we reserved that subject for this chapter. First we'll show you how the muscles should work. Then we'll tell you about various eye muscle problems and how they can threaten vision. Finally, we'll explain what surgery can do to correct these muscle problems —when other kinds of treatment can't be used, or when they fail to work.

As we said in Chapter 2, human eyes work wonderfully and automatically when they are working properly. Without your conscious control, they adjust themselves to changing distances and changing intensities of light; at the same time they work as a team to stay fixed on the subject you're looking at.

Healthy eyes can move up and down and sideways, from left to right and back again, and around. Also, they can rotate, so that if your head tilts a bit the eyes stay upright, with the rest of the world. In other words, healthy eyes are something like the gyroscopes in ships and airplanes: even as the ship rolls or the plane banks, the gyroscope stays fixed in space. Similarly, when eyes are fixed on something, they stay there, even as the rest of your head moves. Consider, for instance, how the eyes of a sharpshooter on horseback stay sighted down the rifle at the target.

This aiming of the eyes at an object and viewing it from two slightly different perspectives gives human beings stereoscopic vision and the ability to perceive depth. It takes a complex system of control to achieve this; in fact, the system is so complex that we won't go into all of the details here. Instead, we'll touch on some major points of this system which you need to understand.

One important factor is the brain. It controls eye movement on the basis of the information transmitted to it—much as you would control a remote television camera on a closed-circuit system, such as you might use to survey a store. For instance, when two healthy eyes are looking at an object (such as this: +), the brain will "see" two images (like this: + +), one from each eye, and put them together into one combined image (+). Eye experts call this *fusion*. Now, the brain will attempt to move and control the eyes so that identical images fall on identical portions of the retinas. This means, for instance, that as objects get closer to you, your eyes have to aim more and more inwards toward your nose. This is called *convergence*. (At the same time, of course, your brain is also controlling the lens and iris to maintain focus and light level.)

This perfect coordination of the eyes in health does not just happen. It's a habit that must be learned. You've no doubt seen a new baby's eyes and noticed its awkward attempts at grasping something, only to knock it over, or to miss it completely. If you've studied an infant's eyes, you've seen both look off in separate directions. It takes about six months for a baby's eyes to become coordinated. By the age of one year, coordination should be pretty well established. Between one and four years, the automatic system will be learning to make minor adjustments, since the ability of the eyes to see (*acuity*, as doctors term it) improves during these early years of growth. At four years, the child's eyes will usually see and work as well as they ever will during his lifetime.

As in most learning processes, there are rewards for accomplishment. Here it is the satisfaction of being able to grab a block when the child wants it, of not running into a wall, or of touching its mother when she is near.

Involved in controlling the movements of the eyes are some other inputs to the brain besides the images which the eyes see. The inner ear plays a key role here. It may seem strange to you to find there is a linkage between your ears and eyes. But if you think about it, and then gain a few facts, you can easily understand the reason for the connection. For instance, you instantly and reflexively turn your eyes and head toward noise, a loud sudden sound you hear, in order to locate its annoying source.

The inner ear is the seat of your sense of balance and, as such, it detects gravity and motion. Turn your head quickly to the right, and your eyes will as quickly turn in that direction, thanks to inner ear information. Also, if your head tilts up or sideways, your inner ear sends to the brain signals which result in the eyes maintaining their position in space. When your eyes give you information about the uprightedness of the world which does not agree with the information from your inner ear, the result is dizziness and nausea. This occurs in certain diseases such as Meniere's.

There are also some inner controls to eye movement. When your eye moves as far as it can up or down, right or left, your neck will then turn in the direction in which you want to see. When you sleep, your eyes roll up; this is called Bell's phenomenon.

You can override your brain's automatic control of healthy

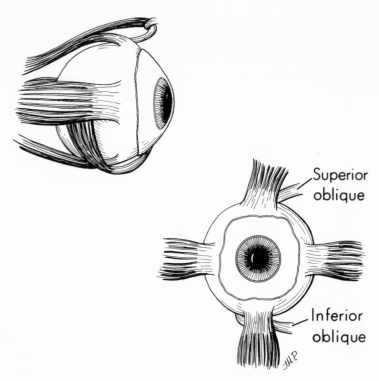

FIG. 2. Extraocular Muscles. Six muscles move the eyeball. Four rectus muscles produce vertical and horizontal motion. The superior rectus turns the eye up; the inferior rectus, down. The lateral rectus turns the eye away from the nose; the medial rectus, toward the nose. Two oblique muscles keep the eyes vertical when the head tilts a bit. The superior oblique runs through a ring of cartilage on the nose.

eyes, to some extent. For instance, you can wilfully move your eyes this way and that. But you should not normally be able to "unlock them," that is, make one look right and the other left. If that occurs, something is wrong.

All of the motions of an eye are accomplished by six muscles, called the *extraocular muscles* because they are located outside of the eye (as opposed to the iris and ciliary body which are inside the eye). There are four *rectus* muscles, one attached to each side and one to the top and bottom of the eyeball, about a quarter of an inch or half a centimeter from the cornea. Depending on their location, these act to rotate the eyeball upward, downward, right and left. Each eye has another pair of muscles which, when they pull against one another, act to rotate the eye like the steering wheel of a car. These are the *oblique muscles* which are attached to the eyeball behind the outside rectus muscles—that is, behind the right rectus in the case of the right eye, and behind the left in the case of the left eye. The upper or *superior oblique* muscle is additionally fascinating because it uses a pulleylike ring of cartilage that juts toward the eye from the nasal bone.

Keep in mind the fact that each muscle is far stronger than it needs to be to move the eye. In fact, only about one percent of the fibers of each muscle work to move it at any time. This is one reason that healthy eyes can be used for so many hours without showing signs of fatigue. Also, these muscles are attached to the eyeball at points where they can effect the most motion with the least force.

It is normal in healthy eyes for one to be somewhat dominant over the other; in other words, people are right- or left-*eyed* just as they are right- or left-*handed*. This means that one eye is usually used as the sighting eye—to find and look at an image—and the other eye follows by converging and focusing on it. The sighting eye is the one a person relies on when shooting with a gun or a camera or when sculpting, drawing, or painting from life. An easy way to tell which eye is dominant is to quickly point your finger at an object. Without moving that finger, close one eye and then the other. The eye that is fixed on the finger is dominant; when you close it and look at the finger with the other eye, the finger will appear to jerk and move over. Right-handed people are usually right-eyed.

There are, however, instances in which one eye becomes so dominant over the other eye that serious vision problems result. We'll discuss these in a few paragraphs.

So far, we have told you how a normal and healthy pair of eyes work together in harmony as a well-coordinated team. But, as you know, this does not apply to all pairs of eyes. A U.S. Public Health Service survey reported in 1972 that 1.6 million American school children (about 7 out of 100) have an eye muscle imbalance problem known as *strabismus*. (Many adults have it as well.) Simply put, strabismus is a failure of the eyes to be properly aligned.

Sometimes the misalignment is so noticeable that the person is called "cross-eyed." That is when an eye turns in. When the eye turns out, the condition may be called being "wall-eyed." When eyes turn in, the doctor calls it *esotropia*; when eyes turn out, this is *exotropia*. Doctors also refer to such misalignment of eyes as *squint*. Sometimes, too, the eyes are misaligned vertically; that is, one is higher than the other. The person with uncoordinated eyes sees two images (as + +), called *diplopia*. The images may be so diverse that the brain cannot fuse them into one image. The force of dominance then succeeds as the brain seeks the easiest, least confusing way out. It relies more and more on the image from the dominant eye and suppresses more and more the image from the weaker eye.

In adults, eyes can become uncoordinated and double vision can result after muscle-weakening diseases, including myasthenia gravis, multiple sclerosis, stroke, or from a brain tumor, a cataract, or mucus from an infection. The effects of dominance on vision then depends on a person's age and the severity of muscle weakening and on how well each eye sees—whether with glasses or not and, if with glasses, what degree of correction is needed. In some adults, too, a muscle weakens with age and turns too far, especially when tired.

Sometimes, if both eyes see well and require little lens correction, a person with a disease-weakened eye muscle will see two images of the world for the rest of his or her life. If the unaffected eye also happens to see better than the weakened-muscle eye, the better eye probably will be relied on more and more and become so dominant that the weakened eye actually starts deteriorating as a result of the inhibition imposed on it by the brain. It is as though it physiologically withers from lack of attention.

Deterioration of the unaligned eye and eventual blindness is far more certain to occur in young children with strabismus. The result frequently is *amblyopia ex anopsia* (blindness caused by roving or "lazy" eye). According to some authorities, amblyopia is the most important cause of preventable blindness. Some two million Americans have lost vision because of amblyopia.

There are several causes of amblyopia, but lack of proper muscle coordination in early childhood is the most frequent cause. If the "lazy eye" is suppressed during the early years of childhood development, it will receive less and less stimulation of light and get "lazier" and "lazier." Like muscles and other organs of the body, the eye must be continually stimulated during the growing years if it is to grow properly and fully. If the eye is not stimulated during these years then, like a muscle which is not exercised, it will wither and deteriorate with disuse.

Children do *not* outgrow crossed eyes, double vision, or amblyopia. If the condition does not receive prompt medical attention, the eye will lose its capacity to see and the child will see with only one remaining eye. According to one survey, 100,000 American children pass this point of no return *every year*. Surveys of U.S. Army recruits and of children living in a suburb of Philadelphia showed that two percent were blind in one eye because of amblyopia. If you are the parent of such a child, the fact that you are reading this book indicates you are aware of your child's problem and will arrange for proper treatment to prevent such blindness.

Not all eye doctors agree on the age limit after which treatment for amblyopia is ineffective. Some say it is four years of age; others say six; still others, eight; while some doctors believe that children with amblyopia can be helped even in their teens. Certainly, each case is different and must be treated in response to its particular and unique needs. It is also certain that the earlier the muscle imbalance is detected and treated, the better the chances for normal vision. This is one reason that the National Society for the Prevention of Blindness, the U.S. Public Health Service, the American Association of Ophthalmology, the American Academy of Ophthalmology and Otolaryngology, the American Optometric Association, and other health organizations stress the importance of thorough eye examinations before a child starts kindergarten, or even before entering nursery school. The nature of muscle imbalance usually is so insidious that the child does not know to complain and the parent has not noticed any problem.

If the doctor suspects amblyopia after examining your (or your child's) eyes, he will conduct even more extensive tests to try to determine the cause. While this chapter is devoted to explaining the needs and techniques of surgery of the eye muscles, you should understand some of the other possible causes of amblyopia and strabismus, and their treatments.

Sometimes there is a tremendous difference in the way both eyes see. One eye may be normal, or require only mild correction with glasses, while the other eye needs a very heavy correction. If this eye is very farsighted, it will turn inward, in order to get the lens to focus, while viewing near objects. This is the automatic convergence-accommodation reflex action we discussed earlier in this chapter and in the previous chapter. If proper corrective glasses are worn to help the lazy eye, it will start to come back to its proper and coordinated position. Sometimes, when eyes are at different levels, other kinds of glasses are used; these have a prism effect so as to bring the image to the cornea, instead of the cornea having to be turned to the object being looked at.

Often, the good eye is covered with a patch, or eyedrops are used to dilate the pupil and relax the lens to keep its images out of focus. The idea of patch and drops is to curb the good eye's dominance over the weaker eye. Then, heavier use of the weaker eye will stimulate it, as exercise strengthens a weakened muscle, to become stronger and more responsive.

The doctor will examine the eyes after a month or so of such treatment to determine if there has been any progress. Often, the weak eye that has started to straighten will turn in, out, or up again once glasses and/or patch are removed. This indicates that the treatment is working and also that it is going to require many months or several years to acquire proper vision. Think of it this way: the eyes now have to learn how to work properly together, as they should have years ago, during infancy. Frequent check-ups are also necessary to evaluate vision in the patched or medicated eye to make sure it is not suppressed so greatly that it develops problems.

Another kind of treatment that helps is optical exercise to retrain the eyes to work together and to help the child regain fusion, or to develop it for the first time in his or her life. These exercises are called *orthoptics*. Another kind of treatment, introduced in Europe, still somewhat controversial and yet to be proved, is *pleoptics*, the retraining of eyes by stimulating them with light.

Very often, amblyopia is the direct result of uncoordination caused by muscles which are paralyzed or too weak, or which pull too strongly. In such cases, surgery is usually the best, and sometimes the only solution. It is also the best solution in adults with disease-weakened muscles. Eye muscle surgery has sometimes been called "minor eye surgery," but in truth there is no such category. True, eye surgery involves very small parts and requires operating with the use of a microscope, but there is nothing minor about it. Still, it is among the safest and surest of all operations of the eye and of any part of the body.

The surgeon ultimately either weakens or strengthens the pull of the errant muscle(s) of the turned eye. He may be able to do this in one operation; or it may take several operations. Each operation is relatively short in time, typically taking only an hour or two.

All eye muscle operations begin the same way. (To learn how you will be readied for your operation and cared for afterward, see the last chapter.) The eye is stable and relaxed, under the influence of anesthesia. The surgeon makes a curved incision with his precise eye operation instruments, cutting through the mucous membrane (*conjunctiva*) and the layer below (*Tenon's capsule*); he pulls these aside gently, exposing the muscle. Sometimes the surgeon will make the exposing incision just at the muscle, where it is attached to the eyeball; sometimes he will make the incision at the *corneal-scleral junction* or *limbus*—where the clear cornea meets the white sclera.

Thanks to orthoptic tests done before the operation, the surgeon knows exactly how much the eye needs to be permanently rotated, and he uses calipers to measure the distance the muscle needs to be moved. If a muscle is pulling more strongly than it ought to be, he will sever it at its attachment to the eyeball, and reattach it by sewing it back on a fraction of an inch toward the rear. If the muscle is too weak, he'll cut out a small segment and sew it back together, tightened. Often when a *retroplacement* or *recession* (weakening) operation is done on one muscle, a *resection* (strengthening) operation is done on the opposite muscle (such as right-and-left, and upper-and-lower).

After he has altered the muscle, the surgeon closes the covering layers of the eye, sutures (sews) them shut, and protects the eye with a bandage. The bandage probably will be removed in twenty-four hours so that you'll be able to move the eye. The idea is to prevent adhesions from forming; these are attachments of tissue that grow during the healing and scar-forming process which later could interfere with free motion of the eye.

When you look at your eye after surgery, you'll notice

its redness; it probably also will be very sensitive to light. It won't hurt, but will instead feel uncomfortable. Most of the discomfort is caused by the rubbing of your eyelids over the stitches.

Usually, you can sit up the first day, go home in two days, and get back to school or work and most other activities two days later. Three or four weeks later, you can participate in mild activities such as swimming (with goggles, to prevent infection from the pool water), or golf. Any more visually strenuous activities such as ping-pong and horseback should be avoided for longer periods, to prevent jostling of the eye until the transplanted muscle is firmly attached.

It will take weeks for the redness to completely disappear. It will take time, too, for the muscles and nerves to resume their full function. Your doctor may want you to see an orthoptist regularly so as to exercise the muscle until it learns proper action and coordination. After the operated muscle has healed, the doctor will measure the eye's movements and decide whether another operation is needed on another muscle. As we have said, several muscle operations are not unusual on an eye, even in tots.

There are other kinds of muscle operations besides those we've mentioned. Sometimes, if a muscle is pulling too strongly for reasons not of visual habits or development but because of emotion, the doctor may prescribe a muscle relaxant. This was the case with baseball star Ernie Banks, who started missing the ball because a convergence muscle tightened into spasm from tension. Other times, the surgeons will simply sever a muscle and not reattach it (*myectomy*). In the case of a too-strong or spastic oblique muscle so treated, the other five muscles can take over and move the eye more normally. Conversely, if a muscle is paralyzed or very weak, the surgeon can reattach it and considerably strengthen it or can strengthen nearby muscles to take over its function.

Sometimes *trauma*—a severe blow—can seriously injure eye muscles. Carmen Basilio's eye muscles (see Chapter 1) were so heavily traumatized that they bled. The outer coatings of the eye had to be opened so the blood clots could be removed and the torn muscles stitched so they could regain their full strength again.

After your muscle operation(s) and retraining, your eyes should achieve the kind of coordination that gives you vision such as you've never had before.

4. Cornea Operations

The healthy cornea of the eye is its window. Facing forward, the cornea captures the light of the environment and sends it to the crystalline lens behind to be formed into a sharp image so the eye can "see."

As we explained in Chapter 1, this dome, a half-inch in diameter, is the only transparent portion of the outer covering of the eye. In fact, the cornea is just about the most transparent tissue in the body, even though it is fairly thick—just under a millimeter (about 0.03 in.). One reason is that its five layers of cells are arranged regularly and in parallel rows, so as to provide the least resistance to light. Also, it is bloodless, unlike the rest of the "skin" of the eyeball, which has white pigment and a dense network of blood vessels so as to create the dark chamber in which images are formed. At the *limbus* line, where clear cornea meets white sclera, blood vessels loop back.

The cornea does not feel heat or pressure, but it is exquisitely sensitive to cold and pain. Most people don't appreciate this because the upper eyelid is continually sweeping past the cornea, much like a wiper across a windshield; when the cornea hurts, they instead feel it as something in the eye, along the inside of the lid. (However, when something foreign is imbedded in the cornea, the eyelids don't hurt when open.)

Despite the protection of the eyelids and the bony brow, the cornea, facing front as it does, is vulnerable to many things that come flying at it through the air. Among these are dust particles, ashes, metal fragments; larger objects such as golf balls and knives; and droplets of liquid such as water, hairspray, acid, and alkali. Being soft, the cornea is very easily scratched, or abraded, by dust or soot or eyelashes that become lodged inside a lid or behind a contact lens, or by fingernails or the twigs of trees that may scratch across it. Sometimes, the injuring metal particle or soot actually will become buried in the soft, clear tissue of the cornea. Sometimes, the cornea is scratched so deeply that it is torn (*lacerated*) to the degree that the aqueous humor (or, simply, aqueous), the watery fluid under it, seeps out.

Under the right conditions—mostly rest and cleanliness —the cornea can do a fairly good job of repairing itself. Unfortunately, in many instances, things go wrong and loss of sight is the result. In fact, according to The National Institute of Neurological Diseases and Blindness, corneal injuries and ulcers are responsible for ten percent of the blindness in America.

One thing that can go wrong is scarring, which comes about as the cornea tries to heal itself, but not successfully. Abrasions which damage only the outer layer of the cornea, the *epithelium*, usually heal successfully because this can regenerate and grow new tissue. The eye should be forced to rest at that time by covering it with a patch for a day or two to accelerate healing. But if the injury goes deeper, scar tissue forms in the healing process—and that is always opaque.

The tolerances here are very tight. The epithelium is only

five cell layers thick, so it can be penetrated by sharp objects or corrosive chemicals. The corneal window through which we see our world and the universe beyond is but a fifth of a square inch in area per eye and we use only the fraction in front of the pupil! So any opacities, no matter how slight, can seriously interfere with vision.

Thin though it is, the outer layer of the cornea is usually an effective shield. The slightly antiseptic action of the tears helps somewhat, but not completely, to ward off molds, bacteria, and viruses that are wafted by air currents, and which may reside deep in the folds of the conjunctiva, under the upper and lower lids.

Once the shield is pierced by a sharp, even though microscopic, object, the germs can get in and gain a foothold. Not having a direct supply of blood containing germ-fighting forces, the cornea is temporarily defenseless against these microorganisms; their foothold in this nice warm and moist medium can rapidly grow into a serious infection. Often the germs, as they inflame and irritate and infect the cornea, destroy cells and produce small areas of erosion known as *ulcers*. Unchecked, the marauders often can eat completely through the cornea in what doctors call a *perforating ulcer*.

Once the cornea is inflamed (a condition medically known as *keratitis*), the tiny blood vessels that loop at the limbus swell with blood and become visible as a halo of radiating red hairlines. Then large numbers of the defensive elements of the blood such an antibodies diffuse into the cornea and battle the infectors.

The pain from such infections, especially if they come as the result of injury, is incredibly sharp (as you may know). Sometimes the body's natural forces will successfully curb the infection and it will subside. Other times, the eye surgeon will have to be called to help. He may simply prescribe antibiotic ointments or drops that have to be put in the eye several times a day. Or he may (as is often the case with *herpes simplex* viral infection) have to scrape away the damaged cells and drop an iodine medicine into the eye. This is done under local anesthesia, of course.

Herpes simplex, incidentally, is one of the most insidious kinds of infection of the cornea. Children often get it when an adult who harbors this virus (which is also responsible for cold sores) kisses them near, or on, the eye. This virus is the most common infectious source of corneal ulcer-caused blindness.

Herpetic keratitis, as the condition is called, is often not recognized for what it is, despite prolific tearing, light sensitivity, and pain. Sometimes little "cold sore" pimples form around the cornea, but more frequently branching twiglike lines called *dendritic ulcers* are etched in the cornea. The eye doctor will look for this with the help of *fluorescein drops* to make the cornea glow under ultraviolet light.

If the herpes is caught in time and treated by scraping, freezing, iodine, or by a unique modern antiviral drug nicknamed IDU (for 5-ido-2-deoxyuridine), it can often be stopped while it is still in the epithelium. If not, it can worsen and become *disciform* or saucer-shaped and deep.

Infection by *herpes zoster*, the virus of shingles and chicken pox, is even more dangerous. Despite treatment, the infection usually leaves the effects of its pox on the cornea. (Antibiotics and sulfa drugs are useless, since they only combat bacteria, and this herpes is caused by a virus.) Shingles, as you may know, starts at the spinal cord and works its way along nerves around and to the front; as it does so, it traces a line of red pimples in the skin. A clue to its involvement of the eye is a pimple on the tip of the nose or the upper lid.

Bacteria and molds also cause dangerous and sometimes even more destructive ulcers of the cornea. As these germs infect, they form *serpent ulcers*, called this because of the way they start as a gray spot and advance in a line toward the center of the cornea. If the infection is unchecked, the ulcer can creep down through the cornea, affect the iris below and leave a pool of easily seen yellowish pus underneath the cornea (*hypopyon*).

As mentioned earlier, such infections are often the result of a dirty foreign body scratching across or lodging in the cornea. Sometimes, though, there is no injury; germs instead come from elsewhere in the eye, such as an infected tear sac at the nasal corner of the eye. The bacteria most dangerous to the eye are *pneumococcus*, *pyocyaneus*, *streptococcus*, *staphylococcus*, and *diplobacillus*.

Some of these bacterial infections are so severe that they can destroy a cornea in a week or so. That is why early antibiotic treatment is essential. While fungus infections are typically much slower in their spread, the same principle applies: the sooner they are treated with antifungal medicine, the better.

Germ-fighting medicines sometimes are given *systemically* as pills or injections, but are usually given as eyedrops or ointments. You can easily learn to drop the liquid medicine into your eye by tilting your head back, staring at a spot on the ceiling and taking careful aim with the eye dropper exactly above your eye. You don't have to hit the dead center of your eye; anywhere between the lids is OK; the medicine will spread over the cornea with the first blink, and you should keep your eye closed for two or three minutes after. Ointment is a bit easier to use. You squeeze some from the tube to your *very* well-washed and well-rinsed fingertip, then turn it into the outside corner of your eye; when you blink you'll notice a haze which indicates the ointment is spreading across your cornea. Of course, having your spouse, parent, or friend do it is even better.

In some cases, especially when the infection has invaded, or is in danger of invading the iris, the doctor may instead inject an antibiotic under the cornea. He'll do this in the hospital or in his well-equipped treatment room, anesthetizing the eye first. He may use the needle to suck out any pus that may have accumulated, and with it some of the contaminated aqueous humor in the anterior chamber of the eye. Or he may make a slit at the edge of the cornea. The eye will quickly replace this watery fluid, incidentally. He'll send a sample of the pus to the laboratory for analysis and for a sensitivity report so he'll know which antibiotics are most effective—hopefully the one he has started with.

In rare and very serious instances, the surgeon may cut through the cornea just ahead of the advancing edge of the ulcer, just as firefighters create firelines ahead of forest fires to halt their advance. In both instances, this is a rather drastic action. Medically, this is known as *delimiting keratotomy*.

Incidentally, one of the most serious infections of the cornea we haven't yet mentioned is caused by congenital syphilis. Once rare, this is becoming more common with the spread of venereal disease, especially among young people of childbearing age. The syphilitic baby may be born with infection in the deep tissues of the cornea that causes what is known as *interstitial keratitis*. The whole cornea, not just an ulcer, is affected.

Besides infection, there are other causes of corneal problems that require treatment, including surgery. Some are due to nervous and metabolic problems, others to lack of tears. Allergies also can cause corneal inflammations. Usually the conjunctiva is also inflamed and the inflammation is seasonal, related to pollens or molds. Ointments with cortisone-like medicines can bring relief, and desensitizing injections over many months may be necessary. Sometimes, the allergic inflammation is not due to anything in the air, but is a reaction to a food, a medicine, or even to an infection.

Allergies may also be an indirect cause of another kind of cornea problem. Technically known as *keratoconus*, it is a cone-shaped cornea. Dr. Frederick Ridley of London, who has studied hundreds of such cases, says three out of four cone cornea cases have such allergic conditions as hay fever, asthma, and skin rash. The allergies cause itching of the eyes, which is met by rubbing with the hands. This continual

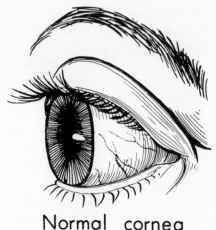

Normal cornea

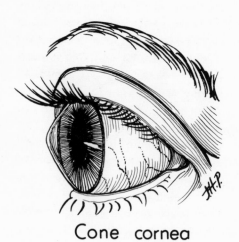

Cone cornea

FIG. 3. **Keratoconus.** This cone-shaped distortion of the cornea can be clearly seen when the eye is in profile. Its severe distortion causes extreme nearsightedness with astigmatism. If the pointedness progresses, it may actually break at the apex.

pressure of rubbing of the eye, especially over the cornea, causes it to deform, in the British doctor's view. He reported that by stopping the itching or the rubbing, he has been able to cure or halt keratoconus.

In late 1972, an American doctor who had immigrated to Florida from Cuba, reported that he had another kind of treatment for keratoconus. Dr. Antonio Gasset of the University of Florida found that high heat (about 332° F.) applied quickly to the cornea could change its shape. By proper application, he was able in 10 patients to change the corneas' cone shapes to round ones.

Actually, eye experts don't agree universally with either Doctor Ridley or Doctor Gasset. They do agree, however, that keratoconus frequently begins at about ten years of age or so and is first noticed as nearsightedness with astigmatism. Often one eye develops the condition before the other, but usually both are eventually afflicted.

At first, the eye looks normal, but as the cornea becomes more distorted its cone shape can clearly be seen by looking at the eye in profile. An eye doctor can sometimes detect keratoconus in its early stages with a slit lamp. This clever device sends a vertical line of light slicing into your cornea. The light that is reflected back is in essence an illuminated cross-section. The ophthalmologist will examine this reflection very closely with a binocular microscope from just inches away. One clue the doctor will look for is the *Fleischer ring*, a thin brownish or greenish band in the top layer of the cornea. Another clue is extreme thinning of the cornea at the center, where the apex or point of the cone pushes forward.

Distortion of vision is just one of the effects of cone cornea. If the cone continues to increase its pointedness, it may actually break at the apex. The cornea will repair the break with its incredibly able healing properties, but leave a permanent scar, which will seriously interfere with vision.

Sometimes, when the shape of the cornea stabilizes and stops changing, a special contact lens can be used to restore vision. The optics of the lens cancel the distortion of the cornea's bizarre shape. The special lens has to be made with the help of molds of the cornea so that it will perfectly fit the conical contours. This is not the same kind of contact lens which some nine million wearers wear, floating on a layer of tears over the cornea. Rather, this is much larger; it fits over the cornea but also over much of the sclera, as well.

Because cone cornea usually is the kind of degeneration which doesn't stabilize, contact lenses may be only a temporary measure. A more permanent solution for most people with keratoconus is surgery—in most cases, a corneal transplant, which we'll describe in detail below.

Cone shape is but one of a galaxy of degenerative corneal conditions. Some of these conditions are considered to be effects of the aging process, perhaps due to the clogging of tiny blood vessels and the subsequent interference with proper supply to the cornea of necessary nutrients from the blood. Other conditions (called *dystrophies*) are the result of some inborn errors which are inherited; some are evident in infancy, but others do not occur until much later, even in the teen years.

Finally, a large number of cornea problems are due not to any disease, but to injury. We have already mentioned the fact that dust and pointed objects frequently scratch and pierce the cornea. Many corneas are destroyed not only by such flying hard objects but also by flying droplets of corrosive liquids, such as battery acid and drain cleaner. Often such accidents take place on the job, but many also occur in sports activities and at home. The result of such chemical burning of the cornea can be scarring and clouding and even the growth of blood vessels over the cornea.

Corneal transplant, one of the wonders of modern surgery, is the answer to many permanent problems of the cornea. While the first human corneal transplant was successfully performed at the beginning of this century, the technique was not available to most people who needed it until midcentury. Even at that, it ranks as the first successful kind of transplantation in the human body.

Also known as a corneal graft or *keratoplasty*, the operation was kept in the dark for generations, mainly because doctors could not believe that living tissue could be transplanted from one human body to another and survive.

As far as we can tell, Alois Glogar, an Austrian workingman, was the first human being to benefit from a corneal homograft (transplant from another person). Actually, corneas had been transplanted to both of his eyes, but only one took. The man who gave him his sight was Dr. Eduard Zirm, who performed the operation on December 7, 1905. The transplants came from the eyes of a child who had just died. Doctor Zirm later reported, "I presented him to our local medical association. By this time six and one half months had passed since the operation. Yet the implanted cornea was completely transparent. And it has retained that transparency to this day."*

While American doctors wouldn't believe such miraculous surgery possible, Russians pulled way ahead of everyone else. As early as 1912, Dr. Vladimir Petrovich Filatoff of Odessa began routine corneal transplantation (by the time he died in 1955 he had performed more than 1,000), using the corneas of fresh cadavers. It would take two generations for American ophthalmologists to catch up to the Russians. One of us (RAP) performed one of the first successful American corneal transplants in 1939. It came as the result of learning about Filatoff's procedure in 1934 from a Russian doctor on a visit to New York. Back at Northwestern University, RAP duplicated and improved the Filatoff procedure in experiments on rabbits and then convinced the head of the ophthalmology department that the operation could save the sight of humans.

This first corneal transplantation was performed on a thirty-two-year-old woman on November 26, 1939. A chronic eye-rubber, her cone cornea was scarred and there-

*Fred Warshofsky, *The Rebuilt Man*, (New York: Thomas Y. Crowell Co., 1965), pp. 28-29.

fore opaque at the tip. The fresh cornea transplanted into her eye came from the clear eye of a stillborn infant. As soon as the sutures were removed, she went to a movie theater and stayed the entire day, fascinated at viewing what had been previously denied her by her disease.

Further research revealed that Dr. Ramon Castroviejo of New York had been working on corneal transplants since 1932, and J.W.T. Thomas of England had been experimenting on this since 1930. The point is that, except in Russia, corneal transplants had really been around for many decades before the technique was universally accepted and used by eye surgeons.

Corneal transplants could be so successful so early in the twentieth century for two main reasons. One was that in an adult eye, which is fully developed, vision may become very poor as a result of clouding of the cornea, but as long as there is no other disease, the eye can still function. This means that replacing the cloudy window can restore sight. Many people confuse this with the rapid loss of vision in the unstimulated eye of a growing youngster.

The other factor in the cornea's favor is that no blood courses through it. Other kinds of tissue unsuccessfully transplanted during the many attempts over the centuries have profuse blood supplies. The blood provides nourishment to the tissues, but also brings prodigious numbers of white cells and other natural attackers of foreign intruders. The result is what is known as *rejection*, the destruction of the transplanted tissue and, therefore, failure. This was as true in the heroic heart transplants of the 1960s as it was of simpler transplant attempts in the Middle Ages.

But this was not true of the cornea since the blood vessels which serve it detour at the limbus and send only their nutritious fluids on to the cornea. Likewise, the cornea is fed protein and Vitamin C from below by aqueous fluid which circulates in the anterior chamber. The tears which bathe it above contain a mild germ-fighter to help keep infection away.

The transplant operation itself is actually quite simple in concept, though it is exacting in its execution. A circular knife or *trephine* is used much like a miniature cookie cutter to remove a disk of cloudy or misshapen tissue from the center of the afflicted cornea. Then a disk of clear cornea of exactly the same size is trephined from the eye of a recently deceased donor and this is inserted into the hole in the cornea made in the afflicted eye.

The new cornea is not just dropped into place. First hair-thin sutures are sewn into both the receiving cornea and the transplant and then the transplant is gently lowered down. Once the transplant is in proper position, about ten more stitches are sewn around the circle to hold it in place. Each suture, incidentally, is placed with a curved needle which is so sharp it can be used only that one time. Each needle penetrates only the upper half of the 0.8 mm thickness of the cornea. The binocular operating microscope (introduced by RAP in 1946) makes such precision possible. To test his "sewing job," the surgeon may inject a bubble of air under the cornea to be sure it is air- and aqueous-tight.

When the transplant is firmly in place, antibiotic may be placed in the eye, then the lids are closed and it is bandaged. The bandages stay on about a month, and the sutures are removed in three or four months, at the hospital.

There are two theories as to what happens next. One is that new corneal cells grow into the transplant, using it as a framework, and after a while replace it. The other theory is that the transplant continues to live as a separate entity—a *chimera*—in space provided and nourished by the host.

In the early days, an eye transplantation pioneer (RAP), spent many evenings in mortuaries, removing the eyes of newly dead and unclaimed bodies of paupers, then rushing home to place the eyes in a refrigerator for the night for transplanting the next morning.

But today medical centers have eye banks and, thanks to the imagination and energy of Dr. Alson E. Braley, eye surgeon, and Ted A. Hunter, psychology professor, both of the University of Iowa, in emergencies eyes can be provided by the Eyebank Network. Both men were hams—amateur radio operators—so they enlisted the help of other hams to instantly flash requests for eyes around the country. The American Academy of Ophthalmology and Otolaryngology set up communication among eye banks. And the airline and the Red Cross cooperated by speeding the eyes—in special cold containers—from donor locations to recipient locations. Under ideal conditions, eyes are removed within four hours of death and corneas transplanted within twenty-four hours.

You now know that only the cornea, a small portion of the eye, is actually used for transplanting. Many patients don't understand that and think that the entire eye is transplanted. Even at this advanced stage of development of surgical art and sciences that is not possible!

There are new developments to preserve corneas indefinitely. One is the frozen storage of whole corneas being developed at the University of Florida. Another freezes only the top layers of the cornea; this has been under development longer at George Washington University.

About eighty percent of corneal transplants "take" and remain clear. But even with the most scrupulous attention to the details of obtaining the donor eye and preserving it, the preparation of the recipient's eye and the transplant operation, some corneal transplants fail. Sometimes the transplanted tissue can acquire the same disease or condition as the tissue it replaces, especially in the case of inherited or congenital cornea degeneration. Sometimes the original infection isn't completely conquered and invades the transplanted tissue. In the case of alkali burns, sometimes the tissue left in the eye is too damaged to latch on to the new tissue; or the damage spreads into it, clouding the new tissue as it did the old.

For eyes in the small but tragic minority in which corneal transplants fail, there can be second chances. There is promising research, for instance, in the use of enzymes to make alkali-injured tissue more normal and more accepting of grafts. There is also the artificial cornea, a plastic window implanted to replace cloudy natural tissue, as was done in 1973 for labor columnist Victor Riesel. Artificial corneas were tried a century ago, with glass, but not until modern plastics were produced was the concept realized. The most successful implant design looks much like a squat telescope: a cylinder with plastic windows at front and back. The plastic implant, again, doesn't work in every case in which it is needed, but it can bring vision to some people in whom transplants fail.

Speaking of plastic, a contact lens is often prescribed after the corneal transplant has "taken" and healed (and sometimes during healing). For one thing, the lens can provide protection for the transplant. Also, a *soft* contact lens acts like a bandage and in fact can be designed to mete out small doses of helpful medicine such as an antibiotic or cortisone. Another reason for the contact lens is that in the case of cone cornea, the eyeball is frequently elongated so as to be seriously nearsighted.

Not everyone who has corneal problems can benefit from a transplant, but an estimated 15,000 of the nearly half a million blind in the United States can. Around the world, there are perhaps fifty million blind people whose sight could be restored by transplants and who could see roses or other flowers for the first time, as did Clyde in Chapter 1.

5. Glaucoma Operations

Your eyeballs maintain their ball-like shape in rather marvelous ways. As we explained in Chapter 2, the large, dark chamber of the eye is filled with a jellylike substance, and the bright front bulge of the eye is filled with a watery fluid. Under this bulge, the space in front of the iris which you can see is the anterior chamber; the dark chamber between the iris and the lens is the posterior chamber.

These chambers are filled with clear substance, the quantities of which are controlled much as dams control the levels of lakes or reservoirs behind them. The thick vitreous humor is rather stable, being formed once and never renewed. It is contained in a membrane and what little fluid may be lost over the years is replaced by more watery fluids. Under the cornea the situation is different; there is a continual turnover of aqueous humor, or eye water. Produced by the ciliary body (which also controls the shape of the lens), this thin fluid circulates from behind the iris across the front of the lens, through the pupil, and under the inside surface of the cornea.

Normally, about a drop (two cubic millimeters) of new aqueous humor is made a minute. This means that the eye has to let old aqueous humor flow away at the same rate. It does this by a clever drainage system at the base of the cornea. The main part is the Schlemm's canal, a circular collection drain which acts much like the rain gutters around the edges of a roof. Stemming off from this canal are "downspouts" which carry the aqueous humor away to tiny veins in the sclera or "skin" of the eye; then the eye water mingles with the general blood stream.

As a rain gutter can have screening placed over it to keep out leaves and twigs that could plug the downspouts, so Schlemm's canal has a screen called the *trabecular meshwork* to trap dead cells and other microscopic debris. Microscopic strands that make up this mesh crisscross in such a way that aqueous humor drains away through smaller and smaller openings. Finally, after it passes through the mesh, the aqueous humor has to seep through the pores of a layer of cells to reach the canal.

Normally, its flow is a perfect harmony of production and drainage. The aqueous humor provides nourishment to the cornea and oxygen to the lens (which, unlike other tissues of the body, has no blood vessels running through it, as we explained in Chapter 4). It also provides an exceedingly clear medium for transmitting the light gathered by the cornea to the lens; and it produces just enough pressure to support the domelike cornea and help maintain the eye's shape.

Unfortunately, things can go wrong and upset nature's very nice arrangement. For some reason or other, the production of aqueous humor can be altered. Or, the drainage of the aqueous humor can become impaired, and as when the outlets of a dam have been shut, the waters accumulate in the anterior chamber and the pressure rises. The waters are forced into the cornea, causing it to swell, producing a halo effect. Swimmers see these halos, too, and for the same reason—edema, or water accumulation in the cornea. The difference is that in swimmers it is temporary; in glaucoma it is permanent.

The pressure inside the normal eye is greater than inside any other organ of the body. (The very high pressures produced by muscles and bones, which move and lift, are not pressures inside the organs.) Being the extremely sensitive organ it is, the eye can be damaged by too-high pressures. The aqueous humor pushes against the lens and the pressure is transmitted to the vitreous humor, which pushes backwards against the retina and there presses against its delicate and microscopic nerve endings, damaging them. At the same time, the retina is pushed against the next layer, the choroid, squeezing closed its tiny vessels that supply blood and nourishment to the light-sensing nerves.

The nerves first affected are those farthest from the thick retinal artery which enters the eye at the back. This is the reason, if you have glaucoma, that you first lose your side vision; as the glaucoma progresses, your field of vision becomes smaller—like looking backward as you drive through a tunnel.

For centuries glaucoma was confused with cataract. In cataract, the subject of the next chapter, the lens of the eye becomes opaque. It looks milky and gray. Hippocrates, the ancient physician who was the father of modern medicine, coined the term *glaucoma*, which combines Greek terms for "gray" and for "diseased condition." Actually, in advanced glaucoma, the pupil looks grayish, too. A French physician in 1709 discovered that glaucoma is different from cataract.

Glaucoma has been called "the thief in the night" and "the thief of sight" because it usually robs vision in a slow, hardly noticeable way, first in one eye, then the other. Chances are, you didn't consider going to a doctor until something was wrong with your vision. Until then, nothing told you that your eyes were in trouble. Too often, glaucoma is discovered only after its victim has missed a stair and fallen, or has had an automobile accident because he couldn't see.

According to the National Center for Health Statistics,* the vision of 362,000 Americans is impaired because of glaucoma. According to the National Institute of Neurological Diseases and Blindness, an estimated million Americans past forty years of age have glaucoma and don't know it. Glaucoma is therefore a major cause of blindness. The American Association of Ophthalmology states that "every year glaucoma brings blindness to 3,500 more people in the United States. It strikes twenty times as often as tuberculosis." Around the world, an estimated ten million people have glaucoma.

Some people are more likely to have glaucoma than others. Jews seem more disposed to getting *acute glaucoma*, the kind whose onset is rapid. The more common kind, *chronic glaucoma*, seems to run in families by skipping generations, so that brothers and sisters who develop glaucoma will have parents and children who do not. Children of a parent with glaucoma may not themselves have it, but their children might. Twice as many women as men have glaucoma.

Researchers trying to detect clues to find those who inherit glaucoma have discovered they can't stand the bitter taste of the chemical phenylthiourea. If you know you may develop glaucoma you can help prevent its consequences, especially if you start taking the proper medicines early enough.

Actually there are other clues that glaucoma leaves which reveals its presence. You should know them so that you can tell if your condition is changing and, if so, immediately inform your doctor.

Prevalence of Selected Impairments, Series 10, No. 48. Washington: U.S. Public Health Service, 1968.

We already mentioned that glaucoma is usually a slow loss of sight, starting at the edges of your field of vision and progressing toward the center. In ninety percent of glaucomas, the chronic kind, that is usually the only clue. There is no pain. Only afterward you realize that you had been having your eyes checked more and more often and seemed less and less satisfied with your new glasses. You may also look back and recall that you began to have trouble adjusting your eyes to the darkness of movie theaters and cocktail lounges. Some people also start seeing rainbowlike halos around lights. You may also be one of those whose vision fogged and blurred; you may have trouble seeing close up and suffer from watery eyes.

It may interest you to know that this was Vincent Van Gogh's problem. Glaucoma was the reason the impressionist artist painted halos around suns and lanterns; it was also the reason he left the subdued light of Paris in 1888 to seek the brighter climate of southern France and spent his last years in Arles. Other famous glaucoma victims include Pope Pius XII and Eamon de Valera, president of Ireland.

Chronic glaucoma is the result of a faulty drainage system. Somehow, nature's clever plumbing system for letting old aqueous humor flow out becomes clogged. It is the back-up of liquid that causes the pressure that leads to the visual problems. How the plumbing is clogged will determine the treatment, so your doctor will use a battery of tests far more sophisticated than those any plumber uses to exactly locate the clog in the system.

Sometimes the stop-up is at the very beginning of the drainage system in the trabecular meshwork. Researchers have discovered that as age advances, the strands in the mesh seem to thicken, closing down the opening through which aqueous humor flows. Sometimes, bits of pigment flake away from the iris because of inflammation or for other reasons. Or tissue flakes from the lens capsule accumulate. This stops

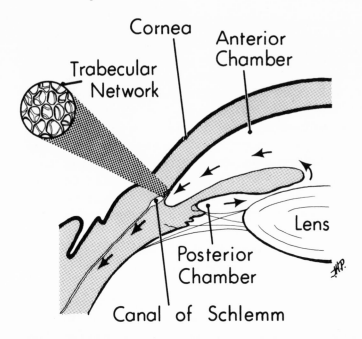

Cornea

Anterior Chamber

Trabecular Network

Lens

Posterior Chamber

Canal of Schlemm

FIG. 4. **Aqueous.** The watery substance in the front of the eye (seen here in cross section) is produced by the ciliary body. It normally flows through the pupil into the anterior chamber, where it helps nourish and support the cornea. "Old" aqueous drains at the base of the cornea via the Canal of Schlemm, and finds its way into the blood circulation.

up the meshwork as leaves stop up the screening over rain gutters, or bits of food stop up the drain of your kitchen sink. (The comparisons, though crude, are accurate.)

Sometimes the clog occurs in Schlemm's canal, which closes down much like hardened arteries or pipes in which rust has accumulated. Or, in fact, the *episcleral veins* which drain aqueous humor away from Schlemm's canal, harden and tighten. Medical studies have shown that people with artery problems are more likely to develop chronic glaucoma than those without such problems. You can see how glaucoma results from aging and understand why people in their sixties are most prone.

The increased pressures are what bring on the symptoms. The increase of pressure forces fluid into the tissues of the cornea, changing its optical properties so as to produce halos and blurring. The pressure against the lens causes other seeing problems, such as inability to focus on close objects.

Chronic glaucoma is often called *open-angle glaucoma* by doctors. This refers to the angle made by the base of the iris and the base of the cornea as they meet, and as seen in cross-section (see Fig. 5). The angle can be measured by a special optical test of the anterior chamber called *gonioscopy*. In chronic glaucoma, the angle is quite open, but in acute glaucoma, the angle is virtually shut.

ACUTE GLAUCOMA

Unlike chronic glaucoma, which develops over a number of years, the onset of acute glaucoma is rapid, with repeated attacks lasting a few hours each. An attack can be so severe and come so suddenly that your family doctor may not realize that your eyes are the cause of your problem. Common symptoms, for instance, are nausea and vomiting (as in appendicitis). Another is a terrific pain in the afflicted eye. Some victims of acute glaucoma have sharp pains in the eye which come and go for a few days before the acute attack. You may even see halos around lights, for a while, only to have them disappear. These *prodromal warnings* are, unfortunately, usually recognized in retrospect, after several acute attacks.

There are other warning signs. Acute glaucoma more usually occurs in small, farsighted eyes. And a *gonioscope* test can cast light on eyes which have shallow anterior chambers and too-acute angles between iris and cornea, which renders the eye prone to glaucoma. This is why acute glaucoma is called *angle-closure* or *closed-angle glaucoma*.

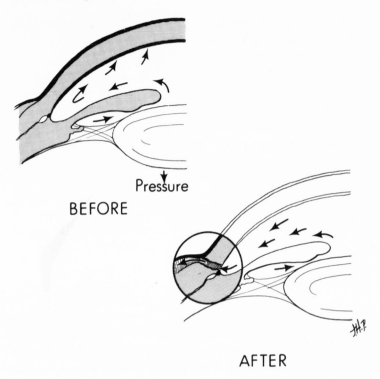

Pressure

BEFORE

AFTER

FIG. 5. Chronic (Open-Angle) Glaucoma. Over the years, the drainage system can become clogged so that "old" aqueous can't leave as fast as "new" aqueous is being made. The result is a build-up of pressure affecting the entire eyeball (as seen here in cross section). One solution is an operation (iridocorneosclerectomy) which allows the aqueous to drain through a hole made in the sclera, or skin of the eye, and under the conjunctiva.

Angle-closure glaucoma is an acute emergency. The base of the iris moves forward and covers the meshwork, cutting off the outflow of aqueous humor. In other words, the drain is plugged. The quick shut-off results in a very rapid build-up of pressure that often goes to three times normal (vs. the 1-1/2 times normal pressure of chronic glaucoma). It is this tremendous pressure forcing fluid into the cornea that pro-

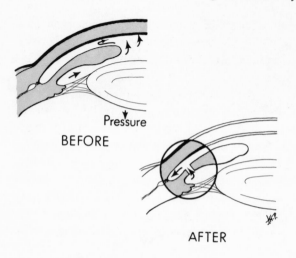

Pressure

BEFORE

AFTER

FIG. 6.   **Acute (closed angle) glaucoma.** Often coming suddenly, and
with much pain, this form of glaucoma occurs when the iris blocks the
free circulation of aqueous. A person with a narrow anterior chamber is
most likely to suffer this rapid increase in eye pressure. Surgery can create
an artificial opening in the iris, through which the aqueous can drain.

duces halos around lights. Also, there is so much fluid in
the anterior chamber that vision becomes foggy. The pressure
inside the eyeball stretches it and produces acute pain and
reddening of the eyes, and, sometimes, swelling of the
eyelids.

Acute glaucoma attacks can be triggered by seemingly
innocent events. For instance, you may walk into a darkened
movie theatre, and as the iris dilates to let in more light it
blocks the trabecular meshwork. You may have consumed
a lot of beer or coffee or other liquids which increased the
amount of liquids in your eye. Having your menstrual period
may produce the same result. As the structures of the eye
swell ever so slightly with fluid, the drainage of aqueous
humor is shut off. So, too, nervous shock or emotional upset
can cause the iris to open and block the meshwork. Typical

was the woman who suffered an attack of glaucoma after a heavy rain in which her basement flooded, ruining her precious den furniture and art. Steroid medicines (related to cortisone), which are sometimes used to treat eye inflammation, can also cause the eye pressure to rise suddenly.

Unless the tremendous pressure is quickly relieved, permanent eye damage with loss of vision results. The pressure causes the same kind of blood cut-off and optic nerve damage as in chronic glaucoma, but it does its damage more quickly. In fact, some victims are literally struck blind in a horror of pain and confusion during an acute attack. That's why the very first attack of acute glaucoma is a medical emergency, like appendicitis, and requires immediate treatment by an eye doctor.

Sometimes acute glaucoma is caused by another eye condition. For instance, a cataractic lens can enlarge so that it pushes forward against the iris and interferes with the flow of aqueous humor. (See Chapter 6.) Or the iris may become inflamed and swollen from irritation or infection and block the normal drainage. When the iris is inflamed it is called *iritis*; when the inflammation is more widespread, and includes the ciliary body, it is called *iridocyclitis*. Sometimes, too, a tumor of the iris near the edge of the cornea moves tissues around so as to stop up the aqueous drainage. A blow to the eye can also cause damage which leads to glaucoma.

You can see that it is very important for an ophthalmologist to examine you as soon as possible so as to determine what is the underlying cause of your increased eyeball pressure. Once he finds the cause, he will know how to treat it.

There is a battery of tests your doctor will perform on your eye if he suspects glaucoma. Some of these tests may be familiar to you; others will seem quite technical and esoteric. Most will not cause you any discomfort; those that do will only temporarily bother you.

The most common test for glaucoma and one that you probably have heard of before, is *tonometry*, or the measuring of the pressure of the eyeball (called *intraocular pressure*). If you are past forty years of age, you should have been given such tests annually by your family doctor. An office eye pressure test takes a few minutes and is painless. The instrument used, called the *Schiotz tonometer*, looks something like a miniature weight scale; but it measures pressure and not weight. Before using it, the doctor will place a drop of analgesic in each eye, and wait a few minutes for it to take effect. Then, while you lie relaxed on your back, he gently holds your lids open with one hand as he delicately and slowly lowers the tonometer onto your eye. You don't feel the plunger in the instrument press against your cornea. It measures eyeball pressure much like a tire pressure gauge. (There is also an electronic tonometer which works so fast that anesthesia isn't necessary.)

If your family doctor has suspected that you might have glaucoma, he has sent you to an ophthalmologist who will, among other tests, measure your eyeball pressure with a more complicated instrument called an *applanation tonometer*. This is more precise because it measures the force necessary to flatten a standard-sized area of the cornea. This test is done as the eye doctor looks at your cornea through a microscope.

Eye pressure is expressed in the scientific unit of millimeters of mercury (abbreviated mm/Hg), which refers to the force necessary to lift a thin column of mercury in a glass gauge. The average reading for persons over thirty years is precisely 19.63. In common use, any reading above 21 mm is considered suspect.

You should realize that eyeball pressure changes not only with advancing years, but also daily and seasonally, and with normal bodily cycles. For instance, as you might guess, a woman's eye pressure will be lower when she is pregnant and during the first part of her menstrual cycle, and higher during the second part of her period. Many people have two daily peaks of eye pressure, at 9 a.m. and at 6 p.m. Also, eye pressure is generally higher in the summer and lower in the winter. A tight collar will raise the pressure and a serving of wine will lower it.

These variations are all taken into account when the ophthalmologist measures your pressure. There is a good chance that he also will give you a *provocative test*, using one or more "tricks" to unmask the glaucoma. He may, for instance, ask you to drink several glasses of water, then measure the eye pressure after elapsed periods of time. He may measure the pressure after you have been in the dark for about an hour, so your pupils open as wide as they can. Or he may give you a medicine which does this. He may massage your eye by gently rubbing it with the tips of his fingers on your lids, then read the pressures.

Caution: be sure you do not touch or rub your eye for about an hour after the tonometry test. With your eye anesthetized, you can seriously scratch the cornea without realizing it, perhaps causing some of the problems described in Chapter 4.

The ophthalmologist will also want to look at the angle created where the cornea and iris meet, as we mentioned earlier. In this test, a special lens is placed over your eye. It is actually a contact lens but a special kind, not the kind worn instead of eyeglasses. It is a large lens which the doctor places under your lids. It is optically necessary because it bends light enough to enable the doctor to see the inner edge of the cornea; normally, the cornea refracts light away from its edges and toward the center or pupil. By casting a thin line of light through the contact lens, the doctor will be able to see the iris and cornea in cross-section, and thus actually be able to measure the angle at which they meet.

The doctor will also use his familiar hand-held *ophthalmoscope* to look into your eyes and examine the retinas. He will particularly look for *cupping*, which could indicate that eye pressures have destroyed a circular area of nerves and vessels around the head of the optic nerve. If so, its appearance is like the inside of a cup. In acute glaucoma, the fluids in the eye are sometimes so cloudy that the doctor can't see the retina.

Finally, the doctor will actually measure your side and blind spot vision with the help of an instrument called a *perimeter*. You place your chin and forehead on special rests. With one eye closed, but fixed straight ahead at a dot, you are asked to tell the doctor (or his assistant) when you see certain objects he holds, as they come into your eye's field of view, usually on a circular bowl of metal in front of your face. As you respond, he marks a special chart of the visual field of that eye. After the test, he has a veritable map of the vision of each eye.

A normal eye does not see a complete circle, but a field oblong in shape. If glaucoma has caused you any loss of vision, it most likely is an enlargement of your blind spot (called the *Seidel sign*). In advanced glaucoma, the blind spot has enlarged in what is called a sickle-shaped area of no vision (or *Bierrum's scotoma*). Unless glaucoma is checked, the damage will progress and the peripheral areas of no vision will spread until you will be able to see only a small tunnel area in the center. In *absolute glaucoma*, there is no vision.

The kind of treatment the doctor gives your glaucoma depends on the cause of the glaucoma. If you have an ordinary case of chronic glaucoma, he will prescribe medicine you drop into your eye. Most likely it will be pilocarpine (*Epicar, Pilocel, E-Pilo, Mi-Pilo*, and *Pilocar* are some trade names). Derived from the young leaves of a South American shrub, it has been used by doctors for a century. It is called a *miotic* because it induces miosis, or contraction of the pupil. Medical scientists aren't sure how pilocarpine reduces eye pressure, but it may be that the narrowing of the pupil acts to open up the trabecular meshwork and let aqueous humor drain more freely.

There are other miotics your doctor may prescribe. Among

them are carbachol (*Carbachol, Carbacel*, and *Carbamiotin*). Even stronger and longer-acting medicines which help the drainage of aqueous homor may have to be used. Among them are physostigmine and demecarium.

There are other kinds of medicines your doctor may have you take, especially those which act to cut back the production of aqueous humor by the eye. Among these are epinephrine eye drops (e.g., *Lyophrin, Epifrin, Epitrate, Glaucon*) and a group of pills taken by mouth and called the carbonic anhydrase inhibitors (*Diamox, Daranide, Oratrol, Ethamide*, and *Neptazane* are examples).

If you have chronic glaucoma, you must take your eye drops or pills regularly. If the instructions say to put one or two drops into each eye every six hours, you should do just that. (See page 44 for the technique.) The instructions are based on the action of the medicine. The idea is to keep the concentration of medicine in your eye as constant as possible—so as to keep the action on your eye as constant as possible. A promising new approach is a bit of soft impregnated plastic placed in the eye each morning which allows small amounts of medicine to seep out all day long.

In many ways, having glaucoma is like being diabetic. For one thing, glaucoma runs in families. Also, you must constantly take medicine to keep the condition under control. If you get sloppy in taking your medicine, you will immediately suffer the consequences. You also have to watch your daily habits. Get enough rest, and eat a well-balanced diet. A glass of wine and cup of coffee with dinner is all right, but if you drink too much beer, coffee, soda pop, or other liquids, you're liable to get in trouble.

It is very important that you *do not* take any other medicines without first consulting your ophthalmologist. The reason is that medicines taken for other reasons—such as for a cold, or nervous stomach, or skin irritation—can work to increase pressure in your eye. Among the worst medicines of this type are steroids such as cortisone and dexamethasone, and belladonna medicines used to relax irritated stomach and colon, as in ulcers, and for hay fever and colds.

If your family doctor prescribes a medicine for you, be sure you remind him of your glaucoma; if you think you can treat yourself with medicine you can buy at a drug counter, don't take it until you consult your ophthalmologist. And *never* take eyedrops unless prescribed by your doctor.

You should also try to avoid getting overtired and try to keep from having emotional upsets. Both of those conditions can worsen your glaucoma by increasing the eye pressure. So can sitting in a dark room too long, as at a double feature.

The medicines you'll be taking for your glaucoma are quite unlike any you've taken before. Be sure you store them properly. If they are to be refrigerated, do so; room temperature will render such medicines less effective. When drops discolor or cloud, they are stale, and should be thrown out or brought back to the pharmacy.

Because the medicines for your glaucoma are potent, there is a chance that they can also provoke undesirable side effects. Medicines designed to help one part of your body may well affect other parts. Sometimes these undesirable reactions are the price you must pay to keep your vision, but you should tell your doctor about any that occur. Also tell him about any other condition you may have, such as a bad heart or kidney disease. A list follows. We won't tell you which medicines can provoke which reactions, because that might be suggestive and your body might unconsciously adopt some of these side effects without your being aware of the psychosomatic cause. Be sure to watch out for:

> abdominal pain
> blurred vision
> chills
> darkening of color of the eyelids of whites
> diarrhea
> dizziness

excess salivation
fast heartbeat
fever
headache
irritability
loss of color of the eyelids of blacks
nausea
poor low-light vision
red eye
skin rash
sweating
twitching
vomiting
wheezing

Since this is a book on eye operations, you may wonder why we've told you everything about glaucoma and its treatment *except* surgery. We did because we felt you should first understand what caused your glaucoma, how your doctor diagnosed it, and how he would treat it. In chronic glaucoma, medicines are almost always tried first. In acute glaucoma, medicines may help for a short while, but surgery is almost always necessary. The doctor will closely monitor the treatment to see that pressure falls and no further retinal damage results.

In both kinds of glaucoma, the purpose of any operation is to improve the drainage of the aqueous, and thereby reduce the pressure of the eyeball. This is the same reason miotics are used; the difference is that surgery produces full-time and permanent drainage relief. Sometimes, too, the surgeon can decrease the output of aqueous humor by destroying parts of the ciliary body. This is most often done by applying electrocautery—a thin and brief burst of electric spark—at the sclera just above the ciliary body.

The most common operation for acute glaucoma is the most simple. It is called *peripheral iridectomy*. A tiny V-shaped notch is cut at the base of the iris; usually this is done so that the notch is located where most people can't detect it. This is at the top of the eye usually covered by the edge of the upper lid. (See Fig. 7.)

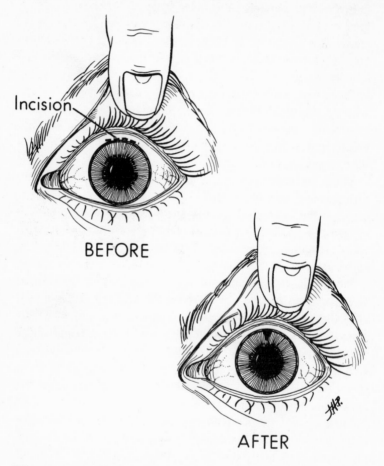

Incision

BEFORE

AFTER

FIG. 7.   Iridectomy. In the most common operation for acute (closed angle) glaucoma, a small opening is made at the limbus, through which a small V notch is cut in the base of the iris. This allows free circulation of the aqueous, thereby reducing its pressure.

There are several ways a surgeon can get at the iris to cut a notch. One is to make a short, curved incision or cut at the limbus, where the clear cornea and the protective membrane that is the conjunctiva meet. The knife creates a small opening to the anterior chamber. When the surgeon pushes gently on the eyeball, the iris pops up. With two snips he cuts a wedge out from the outer edge of that ring of color, then uses a gentle stream of saline solution (mildly salty, sterile water, similar to tears) to push it back into position. He then sutures or sews the layers of the eyeball closed and bandages it.

Since both eyes usually develop glaucoma, some surgeons will operate on both eyes in a "double-header" operation, even if the pressure in the one eye is normal or only slightly greater. Most surgeons will operate on only one eye at a time, unless both eyes are suffering acute attacks.

There are variations on the theme taught and practiced by different eye surgeons in different medical schools, hospitals, and medical centers. For instance, some surgeons prefer to cut the conjunctiva farther away from the cornea, fold it forward, and make an opening in the sclera through which they can reach the iris.

A similar approach often is used for chronic glaucoma. In addition to cutting out a wedge of iris, the surgeon will also slice away a tiny portion of cornea and sclera so that aqueous humor can flow through it out of the eye and under the conjunctiva. This is called *iridiocorneosclerectomy*. In a simpler version, a piece of iris is pulled up into an incision in the sclera and sewn there, to act as a wick to draw out excess aqueous humor. This is an *iridencleisis*.

Delicate as these operations are, there are even more delicate and precise techniques being developed for chronic glaucoma, especially in the Soviet Union, Germany, and England. In one kind of operation, *trabeculotomy*, small cuts are made in the conjunctiva and then the sclera. One more precise incision is made under the guidance of the operating microscope: Schlemm's canal is opened—a remarkable feat considering that it is only 24 microns (thousandths of a millimeter) wide. A tiny wirelike instrument is inserted into the canal and gently flipped to break open the trabecular meshwork at that small portion of the eye. The effect is the same as cleaning leaves out of your rain gutter to let the waters drain away.

Another delicate operation, developed by Prof. M. M. Krasnov of Moscow, is *sinusotomy*. In this operation, a small length of sclera exactly over Schlemm's canal is stripped away, making it an open ditch under the conjunctiva. This is especially useful in glaucomas in which this canal has narrowed and cut off drainage. Prof. Krasnov performed 2,000 of these in the decade 1962-72, with an eighty-three percent success rate. Also being developed is a way to burn a hole in the iris with a laser beam, without the need for a knife.

After you have recovered from your operation, your eyeball pressure will be checked regularly to be sure it has stabilized at a low enough level. There is the small chance that you will have to use medicines to lower it still more, if the surgery has not done the complete job.

Also, your eye doctor will want to check your vision regularly to be sure it has not deteriorated even slightly and even before you are aware of it. In some instances, the effects of high pressure on the retina over a long period of time result in some permanent loss of part of the visual field. Usually, any loss of vision is temporary, but not always. In any case, relieving the high pressure certainly prevents any further loss of vision.

After your glaucoma operation, you'll see and feel better than you have for a long time. And you will be assured that you have been saved from joining the statistics of those who went blind because their glaucoma was untreated.

6. Cataract Operations

If you've looked it up in the dictionary, you already know that cataract comes from the Latin word for "waterfall." It was given this name because it looked to physicians of the ancient world as though a veil of blurry, translucent water had fallen over the lens. Probably because it was so easily seen, cataract was one of the first eye conditions treated by surgeons who began the ophthalmology profession at the dawn of civilization.

Because of this name, many people today believe that a cataract is a film of skin which forms in front of the lens. It is not. Cataract is an opacity of the lens which defeats its purpose of gathering light from the outside world and focusing it into an image on the retina, or back wall of the dark chamber of the eye.

As we explained in Chapter 2, the lens of the human eye is not a solid piece of transparent tissue, like so much biological glass. It is, instead, a living, growing organ. It is made of many layers of cells, much as an onion is. Like an onion, it grows with time; the lens of an eighty-year-old is half again as thick as the lens of a twenty-year-old.

The lens, which has no blood or nerve supply and which is the densest concentration of protein in the body, is unique in still another way. Other tissues of the body get rid of old cells by sloughing them off to the outside world, either directly or through a duct. For instance, every time you brush or rub your skin you shed hundreds of old skin cells. The fact that the uterine cervix sloughs off cells is the foundation of the Pap test; among these may be cancer cells, detected by placing samples of sloughed-off cells under the microscope.

In still other organs, white cell scavengers from the blood roam through the tissues, embracing cast-off old cells and carrying them away for disposal.

Not so the lens. It has no blood supply. It is not exposed to the outside world. It does not open into a body cavity. Instead, the lens retains its old cells. As new cells form on its outside layers, older ones are compressed more tightly toward the center.

Many organs of your body replace their cells many times throughout your lifetime. But in your lens (as in your brain) are the first cells which were formed when you were but an embryo, then a fetus in your mother's womb. These first cells are at the very center of the lens. Around it is a layer of cells deposited in your childhood. Around that is a layer of cells deposited in adulthood. Even now, the lens is adding new layers, getting thicker.

The cells in the center of the lens become compressed, dehydrated, and stiff. This is the main reason the lens loses its flexibility at about the age of forty-two. Something else happens with age: the lens deepens in color as bits of protein accumulate between the layers of cells, from young-adult pale yellow to amber. Also, small opaque bits show up from time to time (these can be seen with a slit lamp).

Aging of the lens interferes with everyone's vision. As you get older you become less tolerant of bright light. Paradoxically, you seem to see better in dim light and to see close objects more clearly. The reason for this is that bright light is diffused by the many layers inside the thick lens; another is that in dim light, and when viewing close objects, your pupils are open wide, thus letting in additional light through the edge of your lens, which is clearer than the center.

Some eye specialists feel that just about anyone who lives long enough will develop cataracts. They base this statement on the fact that the lens keeps losing transparency with age. Still, you have probably read in newspapers or seen and heard reports on television about persons who achieve the age of one hundred years and still can see well, although they may need glasses. The point is, though, that cataract is but another product of the inexorable process of aging, much as are graying of hair, brittling of fingernails, wrinkling of skin, and sagging of breasts. That's why doctors have given it the awful name of *senile cataract*.

Evidence of age's importance is the fact that "for persons 65 years and over," according to the National Health Survey,* "cataracts were reported as the cause of visual impairment in 39.6 percent of all cases—far more frequently than any other cause." This federal survey found that of the nation's million and a third Americans whose sight is impaired by cataract, three-fourths (more than a million) were sixty-five years and older. Another interesting finding is that cataract strikes about twice as many women as it does men.

We are sure that you know that aging is not an isolated factor in diseases such as cataract. The progress of years, by itself, can be innocent. The problem too frequently is that aging works in collaboration with other conditions of the body. For instance, cataract seems to run in families. That indicates that there is some sort of genetic liability involved. In some people the usually faint and slow process which tints the lens instead accelerates and clouds it.

Prevalence of Selected Impairments, U.S. Public Health Service Publication No. 1000-Series 10-No. 48, 1968. Washington: USGPO, 1968. (75¢)

Also, with advancing age, the abuses and poisons which have accumulated over a lifetime begin to show effects on the more susceptible parts of the body. Here, too, genes often determine which tissues of the body these are. As blood circulation becomes impaired, an ever so slight but continual process, not all tissues are fed as fully as they need to be. The lens, without a direct blood supply, still needs to be nurtured. If it does not get proper nutrition, it can form cloudy, abnormal tissue instead of clear healthy tissue.

Also inherited is diabetes, which can cause cataracts not only in the aged but in the young. (Diabetes also causes some of the retinal problems of the next chapter.) Cataracts associated with diabetes are one of the *sugar cataracts*. Diabetes involves the faulty metabolism of the sugar glucose. Sugar cataracts can easily be produced in animals in the laboratory simply by making them diabetic (that is, removing the pancreas, the gland which secretes insulin, the hormone which diabetics lack). Another sugar cataract seen in young children is due to the absence of an enzyme in the liver which converts one kind of sugar, galactose, into the more common form, glucose. (For the technically minded, the missing enzyme is galactose-1-phosphate uridyl transferase.) When *galactosemia* (as the condition is called) is detected in babies shortly after they are born, galactose can be removed from their diets. Otherwise, this sugar will accumulate in abnormal and even toxic amounts in the body. Cataract is one of the results. Xylose is another sugar associated with cataract.

Other kinds of metabolic conditions and diseases, such as arthritis, are associated with cataract, but researchers are not sure exactly what the chemical relationship is. In general, these conditions accelerate the process of lens aging: the fine balance of life processes in the lens tilts the wrong way and protein starts breaking down into its chemical constituents in those newer cells at the outer layer of the lens.

While babies with galactosemia can develop cataracts at a very tender age, there are some babies who get them even earlier—they are born with cataracts. These *congenital cataracts* most often are the result of the mothers'contracting German measles infections during their first three months of pregnancy. (These congenital cataracts often come with deafness.) But there are yet other, unknown, prebirth causes of cataract. There is, for instance, a higher incidence of cataracts among children who are mentally retarded, especially mongoloids. And malnutrition during pregnancy can cause cataracts in unborn children.

Besides conditions inside the body, there are also elements in the external environment which can produce cataract. A drastic change in diet that means absence of certain vitamins or other important elements of good nutrition can cause or provoke cataract just as certainly as a metabolic disease and for similar reasons. So can ultraviolet light, X-ray, infrared (heat), and other kinds of radiation, including microwaves from ovens, radar, and diathermy. (Goggles or sunglasses should be worn when using sunlamps and arc welding or glass blowing equipment, in order to filter out these harmful rays.)

A blow to the eye, and, especially, a sharp object piercing the eye (like a point of metal which flies off a lathe, mill, or drill) can cause a *traumatic cataract*. A very powerful blow can dislodge a lens from the delicate fibers that hold it, and force it back into another position as well as make it cataractous. This is a *dislocated lens*.

Whatever its cause, a cataract is a lens that has become opaque. Usually, the opacity is gradual and advances as slowly as the years, so that members of your family have not noticed, nor have you noticed when looking at your image in the mirror. When the cataract has advanced to the stage at which it severely interferes with your vision, your family probably will be able to see, in bright light, the characteristic bluish-white, silky appearance of the cataract that makes it look like milkglass.

Different kinds of cataracts form different patterns of opacity in the lens. Your ophthalmologist will put drops in your eyes to open your pupils, then illuminate the lens with a slit lamp, which casts a piercing line of light, and peer at it through a two-eye microscope that looks like binoculars. Some cataracts form spots, others form lines which radiate inward from the edges of the lens like the spokes of a wheel; still others form flowerlike and corallike patterns which, under other circumstances, might be aesthetically appreciated.

We mention this because you should understand that the character and pattern of the lens's opacity determines how a cataract affects your vision. Probably, your vision is affected as though someone has turned down the lights—even out in bright sunlight. You may notice that you blink a lot, as in some vain effort to clear the muddiness away from the front of your eyes. You may also notice that the world has a yellow or brownish cast. (You have famous company. This is the explanation given for the muddiness of the water lilies in Monet's later paintings.) With the dimming you may also have noted that bright reflections are annoying because they appear as sharp spikes of light, or perhaps as double rays.

Sometimes, as we mentioned in the previous chapter, cataract comes with glaucoma. Sometimes, too, it comes with retinal problems, as explained in the next chapter.

The treatment for cataract is almost always surgery. Sometimes the doctor can prescribe drops that will help you see. Only rarely can this help, however; that is, when the cataract is very small and near the center of the lens. The drops given are medicines which dilate the pupil (mydriatics such as *Paradrine*) so as to allow light into the edges of the lens and thus "see around" the cataract (but never if you also have glaucoma). Also, in very rare cases, where cataracts are formed at the edge of the lens, special glasses or contacts can be used to direct more light toward the center of the lens. (A fascinating fact of cataract is that in the late stages of development you may find that you can read without glasses. That is, you can focus on near objects even though the level of light in your eyes is drastically reduced.)

The only sure cure for a cataract is its removal. What we mean, of course, is that the only way to get light into your eye is to remove the barrier to that light, which is the cataractous lens. Now, in cataract, as in any other kind of operation on your eye, or on any part of your body, you and your doctor have to reach the decision as to whether and when to operate. It's *your* eye and *your* vision. Jewelers, die makers, tailors, artists and others who require keen vision to work, need the operation as soon as their vision is affected, whereas coal miners, gardeners, or laborers, may hold off having an operation until they barely see at all. When another problem in the eye, like glaucoma, is involved with the cataract, an operation may be quickly needed.

If only one eye is affected and the doctor finds no signs of cataract formation in the other eye, he may want you to come back regularly for examinations. In some cases, especially diabetics, a cataract can develop in mere weeks. Cataracts, especially senile cataracts, can go through four stages. In the first *incipient stage* opacities start to form. In the second, *intumescent stage*, the lens is milky white. In the third, *mature stage*, the lens is totally clouded. In the fourth, *hypermature stage*, the lens has turned to opaque liquid. How fast a cataract moves through these stages depends on many factors, including the state of health of your eye and your total well-being.

Eye surgeons used to wait until a cataract was mature before they removed it. Today, they know this is not necessary. In fact, ophthalmologists recognize that there is a danger in waiting that long. While you may still have vision good enough to get around, your cataract is not going to get better, so you may as well have it out as soon as possible.

There is a real danger in waiting too long. A hypermature cataract can burst, spilling out its contents into the eye and causing dangerous complications.

That's why the decision to have an operation must be a joint decision arrived at by you and your doctor. The cataract has to be removed as soon as it interferes with your doing the things you want to do, and have to do, in daily life; yet it has to be removed no later than the doctor feels is the safe limit.

Cataract removal is the most successful blindness-prevention operation. It is no modern-day miracle, although the instruments used today are new. Cataract removal is an operation which goes back to 1000 B.C. when it was being performed in India by Susruta without a microscope and with comparatively crude instruments. Six centuries later, the operation spread to the Eastern Mediterranean. The first to make the operation known in European surgical circles was a French surgeon named Daviel in 1748.

Today cataract removal operations are about ninety-eight percent successful. Testimony to their rate of success is the staggering statistic of a quarter of a million cataract operations performed in the United States every year. This total represents half of *all* eye operations performed annually in the country.* About eighty-five percent of all persons operated on for cataract achieve normal vision (20/30 or better).

Like other eye operations, the precision which the operating microscope affords produces the best results. It not only enlarges the structures of the eye, but also gives the surgeon added perception of depth. In eye operations, an eighth of an inch up or down is a very big dimension.

In the most common cataract operation, the surgeon makes an opening at the circle (*limbus*) where the clear cornea meets the white sclera. Usually this is done at the top of the eye so it will be covered later by the upper lid. The iris is lifted out and a small pie-shaped cut is snipped (as in glaucoma surgery). This is done to enable the iris to open wide enough for the next step, which is the removal of the yellow jewel that is the cataractous lens. It also assures that the circulation of aqueous will not be disturbed and so induce glaucoma.

Monthly Vital Statistics Report, Vol. 21, No. 3, Supplement (2), 9 June 1972, National Center for Health Statistics, Rockville, Md. 20852.

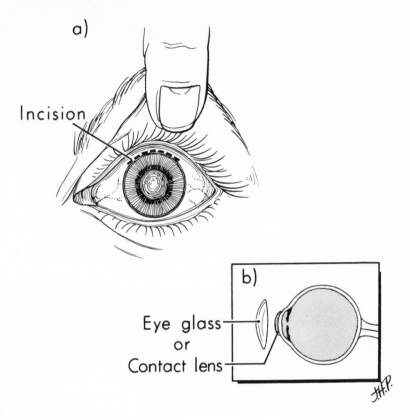

FIG. 8. Cataract Removal. When the lens of the eye becomes opaque and no longer transmits light, it is a cataract. Vision only can be restored by its removal. This is usually done through an incision made at the limbus, from 10-to-2 o'clock. Then the eye needs an auxiliary lens to form an image on the retina. This can either be special cataract eyeglasses or contact lenses.

Now there are variations. Different eye surgeons do it in slightly different ways, depending both on their previous experience and on their patients' problems. Most eye surgeons extract the lens through the pupil. Usually an enzyme (*alpha chymotrypsin*) is used to help dissolve the tiny *zonules* attached to the lens (by which the ciliary body exerts its forces on the lens). Looking through the operating microscope, some surgeons pull the lens out with a tweezers-like forceps, while others use a *cryoprobe*, a small instrument which contains liquid nitrogen in the handle and transmits the ultracold (-195° C.) to a thin tip (or probe) that literally freezes the lens so it comes out cleanly in one solid piece. This technique is called *cryoextraction*. Taking out the entire lens either way is called *intracapsular extraction*.

There is another category of surgery by which cataracts are removed, called *extracapsular extraction*. This means that the capsule, or "skin" of the lens is pierced so the contents can be removed one way or another. In certain congenital cataracts in very young children, and in very old people with hypermature cataracts, the lens substance inside the capsule is watery. The ancient technique which is still occasionally used is *needling*. It is what it sounds like: the piercing of the capsule with the fine point of a needle knife. The old way was to let the watery lens substance leak out and be absorbed by the other fluids of the eye. The new way to do this is to pierce the lens capsule with a hollow needle and mechanically suck out (*aspirate*) the watery substance.

Two space-age versions apply special forces: the unheard vibrations of ultrasound or ultrafast blades (like a kitchen blender) to beat the fibrous senile cataract to a water fluid, so it can be sucked out.

Again, we have to emphasize that different surgeons use different techniques. We can't tell you which one is better than others. One is best for the combination of you, your kind of cataract, and your surgeon's skills.

When the lens is gone from your eye, a tiny void is left behind. The surgeons will fill this with pure saline solution (salt water) to help the eye maintain its ball-like shape and internal pressures. Usually the clear, jellylike vitreous humor which fills the large rear chamber of the eye will stay where it is, since it is contained in a membrane. Then the front part of the eye will extend its watery aqueous humor slightly back to fill in the space where the lens was. Sometimes, though, the vitreous leaks through the membrane and enters the front circulation. This is particularly true in advancing years when the vitreous has become very watery and the membrane weak. In either case, as long as the fluids are clear, vision can be restored.

In only ten percent of cataract patients is only one eye affected. That means that ninety percent of cases like yours require *bilateral* (both eyes) operations. And just as well, in terms of the kind of vision you'll have for the rest of your life. That's why both eyes are usually operated on during the same hospital stay, two or three days apart.

What you have when the lens is removed is an eyeball with only the weak focusing power of the cornea. The lens-less (*aphakic*) eye is much like a camera without an internal lens. The solution to that problem is simple: an external lens, either a spectacle or a contact lens.

You have to face up to the fact that while your vision will be restored and you will be saved from blindness by your cataract operations, thereafter you will be seeing the world differently than before. For one thing, you'll see the world in different colors. It will be brighter. Remember, your cataract probably made your lens yellow-brown, which meant you were looking at the world through amber-colored filters. Now the sky, instead of being a pale blue, will become a deeper color. Also, the objects of the world will be different-sized than before. If only one cataract is removed, this can be a problem, because the images in that eye and in the unoperated eye will be of different sizes. The thick eyeglass lens necessary to help the eye will produce an image which is about a third bigger than the other eye's. This is one reason operations are not always recommended, or are delayed, when only one eye has a cataract, although contact lens make this more possible (see below).

Even if both eyes are operated on, and the doctor pre-scribes glasses, there are some adjustments you will have to make. You'll have to get used to the fact that your coffee cup is not as close to your reach as it looks; it seems closer because it appears larger. Similarly, that step or curb is not as close. Also, the eyeglass creates a distortion which makes doorjambs appear to bow inward and you will wonder whether or not you can make it through. Also, your peripheral vision is restricted, so it is as though you are looking through a tunnel. But if you move your eyes even slightly, the prism effect of these thick lenses gives you a wild version of objects. So, you have to learn to move your head instead of your eyes.

It will take you some time, perhaps a few weeks, to adjust to the world as you now see it through your thick cataract glasses. Just remember that in many ways you are like an infant with new, God-given eyes, learning spacial relationships for the first time. This attitude may, in fact, give you a refreshed new outlook on life (no pun intended!).

If you can wear contact lenses (as do seventy-five percent of cataract surgery patients), you'll be better off. Their magnification is a barely perceptible five percent; furthermore, the lens, since it floats on a film of tears over the cornea, moves with the eyes, making exaggerated head movements unnecessary. This also means there is no distortion when the eye moves off dead-center.

We won't go into the techniques of learning to wear contacts, how you insert them and take them out. Your eye surgeon, optician, or optometrist will teach that to you. Just remember, teenagers can do it for cosmetic reasons, you can do it for reasons of seeing better. Besides, you *may* look better without glasses, even at your age!

Today there are both hard and soft-plastic contacts. The soft lenses are instantly comfortable, but more expensive, and you can only use them if you have no, or low, astigmatism.

Incidentally, some research surgeons have been able to insert special plastic lenses *in* the eye after cataract removal—in fact in the same location as the original lens.

Of course, it can't focus as did the original lens, but in many cases it can be an excellent substitute. However, since the *intraocular* lens is still experimental, it is not likely that your surgeon will recommend it.

7. Retina Operations

The retina is your eye's ultimate sense organ. All of the other structures of the eye—including the cornea, iris, lens, and the aqueous and vitreous fluids—help to cast images of the world's light onto the retina. As we explained in Chapter 2, the retina is like the charge plate of a TV camera, marvelously converting light into electrical signals. Remember, in the case of TV, these signals are broadcast from the station to your home. But your eyes send its signals via the optic nerve to your brain, where you actually "see."

What is perhaps most remarkable about the retina is its gossamer qualities. It seems inappropriately fragile for the crucial role it plays in vision. Only seven-thousandths of an inch (0.18 mm) thick, it stretches across two-thirds of the inside wall of the eye. Its rim is at the front where the ciliary process begins. Though it is tissue-paper-thin, the retina is composed of ten layers of cells. The light-sensitive rods and cones are in the second layer (facing front). By way of various connections, they pass their feeble electrical impulses to the network of nerve fibers in the bottom layer. The retina also has a fine network of blood vessels, which are fed by a central artery that enters at the back with the optic nerve. A central vein lies next to it to drain off "used" blood. (This is but one of its blood supplies, however.)

The inner pressure which the eyeball maintains keeps the retina pressed against the *choroid* beneath it. The choroid serves as a cushion for the retina, and as an auxiliary source of nutrition, even though the many blood vessels of the choroid do not connect with the blood vessels of the retina. In fact, the retina has very few connections at all with the choroid, which is one reason for the problems which we will soon describe. In effect, the retina lies against the choroid like some silky wall covering that is not pasted to the plaster, but is pushed against the wall by the wind.

The retina has the only veins and arteries which are directly visible. By just looking into the eye with a light, a doctor can assess the state of health of the blood vessels of your body. That's why peering into the eye with the hand-held instrument called an *ophthalmoscope* is such an important part of routine physical examinations. Any condition or disease which affects arteries and veins—especially those of the brain—will similarly affect the arteries and veins of the retina. So by looking at the *fundus* or *ground* at the back of the eye, as it is often called, the doctor can gather visual clues as to how your body is aging, whether stroke threatens as arteries harden, if blood pressure is too high, or whether you have diabetes, kidney disease, or a blood condition.

Sometimes when you take a photograph of children with a camera which has an attached flash unit, their eyes will have pink centers. This is the direct reflection of the light of the flash back from their retinas. When the doctor looks into an eye with his 'scope, he sees fine details that look much like a roadmap (see Fig. 9), with veins and arteries radiating out from a hub. This is the *optic disk*, where smaller blood vessels come together to form the central retinal artery, and where nerve fibers come together to form the optic nerve.

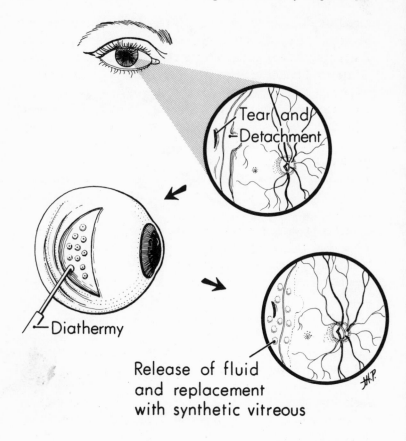

Release of fluid
and replacement
with synthetic vitreous

FIG. 9. **Detached Retina.** Through his ophthalmoscope, the eye doctor
can see wrinkles of the retina which indicate tears and detachments. One
treatment is an operation in which electric heat is applied from the outside
to "spotweld" the retina back in place. Sometimes synthetic vitreous has
to be injected into the main body of the eye to replace that which is lost
through leakage in the tear.

The fundus is a telltale. Its very color, from cherry-red
to milky-white, reveals much. The vessels themselves tell
much, especially if they are thinner or thicker than normal,
or if they twist and turn more than they should.

There are many conditions which can cause these tiny
blood vessels of the retina to leak. Microscopic amounts of

blood which seep out into the vitreous humor will eventually be absorbed by the eye's circulatory system and removed. But in the meantime, the disease can cause damage that often is irreversible and can lead to blindness. (Bleeding can lift the retina away from the choroid, thus ironically depriving it of blood and impairing its function.) When the doctor identifies the disease which causes the hemorrhage—such as diabetes, kidney disease, toxemia of pregnancy—he will act to get the primary disease under control. But he also has to work on the hemorrhage, lest the bleeding cause damage to the retina. Such dangerous conditions of the retina are called *retinopathies*.

Perhaps the most prevalent of these is *diabetic retinopathy*, which is rising in importance as a cause of blindness in industrialized countries. A diabetic is twenty times more likely to become blind than a nondiabetic person of the same age. Researchers at the Harvard School of Public Health late in 1971 analyzed statistics concerning persons already blind from diabetic retinopathy and predicted that by the year 1980 it would overtake cataract and glaucoma to become the leading cause of blindness in the United States.

How likely a diabetic is to develop the retinal disease seems to depend on his or her age when diabetes first appeared and how many years he or she has lived with the disease. Ninety percent of those who found they had diabetes before the age of thirty years and have lived with the sugar disease for more than twenty-five years have been found to have retinopathy. To put it more clearly, if you developed diabetes before thirty and are now fifty-five, the chances are nine out of ten that your eyes have retinopathy!

You can look at this philosophically. In 1921, before insulin became available to all diabetics who needed it, only eight percent of them developed diabetic retinopathy—because most diabetics died at an early age!

In diabetic retinopathy, the tiny blood vessels of the retina undergo changes, as do blood vessels in other parts of the body. The difference is that in the small world of the eye, even microscopic occurrences become magnified into problems that are big and dangerous. A small leakage of blood from your gums means little, for instance. But that same amount of minute hemorrhage in your eyes might lead to blindness.

Diabetic retinopathy can do its damage over a span of two or three years, during which time you feel nothing and probably see nothing different. Then, you begin to notice impaired vision. Your eyesight seems to get worse and worse. Objects are not as well defined as they used to be.

Actually, unknown and unfelt, a disease has been progressing. The walls of the arteries and veins have thickened, interfering with blood flow. This has led to some starving of the retinal tissues, and their collection of watery fluid, which in turn stimulated the growth of new arteries and veins, a process known as *neovascularization* or *vascular proliferation*. Bleeding often occurs at this stage, for several reasons, researchers believe. For one thing, the tiny new blood vessels can grow into the vitreous humor, which, paradoxically, causes this jellylike material to pull away. This severs some of the microscopic arteries, so they bleed. Also, a new surge of blood through the retina to those areas which were previously starved, causes some capillaries to balloon into aneurysms, like the bulge at a weakened spot in an auto tire or a long balloon. These tiny aneurysms, because they *are* weak spots, can pop, releasing blood as they do.

Diabetes usually causes retinal bleeding in middle-aged and older persons. Another condition which can cause bleeding in the eyes in infants was responsible for an epidemic of blindness in the 1950s. The epidemic occurred among premature babies who were placed in incubators into which 100 percent oxygen was pumped. The idea was that the tiny infants needed oxygen, so the more the better. After all, 100 percent oxygen is used with adults with such respiratory ailments as emphysema and pneumonia.

Unfortunately, the oxygen-rich air the babies breathed

caused the arteries and veins in their retinas to tighten. But once these infants were taken out of the incubators and placed in the newborn nursery where they breathed normal air, their retinas became starved for blood and new blood vessels grew quickly to bring in the vital blood. With new pathways created, the blood rushed in, causing hemorrhages and the growth of fibrous tissue. The result is what doctors call *retrolental fibroplasia*. In effect, a scar forms over the retina so that images cannot reach the rods and cones.

Often when the retina bleeds long enough without being treated, another condition, *retinal detachment*, can develop. Remember, a little earlier in this chapter we explained that the retina is not connected to the choroid below, but is held against it by the pressure of the vitreous humor. If blood or anything else works its way behind the thin retina, it acts to push the retina away from the choroid. When that happens, the retina is deprived of one of its sources of nutrition, nerve connections are stretched and it begins to suffer.

People who have suffered detached retinas say they see flashes of light, or a "cloud" across their field of vision, or a curtain being drawn. This can happen immediately, or even weeks after the detachment occurs. There is little warning otherwise. Despite the fact that there is a tear, you feel no ache or pain, nor are you suddenly "struck blind." You may find that you see better in the morning; this is because the retina may flop back into position while you sleep.

Hemorrhage is only one reason why retinas may detach. An even more common cause is trauma, meaning a blow to the eye or the head. This can occur when you bump your head, get hit in a fight, are hit with a snowball or other hard ball, or even during a sneeze. The blow causes the retina to tear, which allows vitreous humor to push through the hole and float the retina off the choroid.

Of course, not everyone hit in the eye or in the head suffers a detached retina. Those who do have some sort of weak spots in their retinas which already existed. People who are nearsighted and thus have elongated eyeballs have been found to have such weaknesses in their retinas. Aging is another factor. Over the years the vitreous humor shrinks. Sometimes as it does so, it pulls the retina with it, away from the choroid. This also occasionally happens when a cataract is removed, especially if it was attached to the *hyaloid membrane* containing the vitreous.

Sometimes, too, cysts or tumors form under the retina and push it out. One of the worst is *retinoblastoma*. (See the next chapter.)

In most instances, your ophthalmologist will be able to see your retinal problems by looking into your eye with an ophthalmoscope. If the vitreous humor is clear, the detached retina will look like loose wallpaper. However, if there has been a lot of bleeding, the vitreous humor may be too cloudy. Likewise, if you also have a cataract, he won't be able to see because that will block the light. If he suspects a detached retina, an ultrasound scanner can be used, like radar in a fog, to find the damage.

With the ophthalmoscope, the doctor will be able to directly see the retina's blood vessels and any hemorrhage, as well as such telltale signs as spots that look like small puffs of cotton. He may use other tests to measure your fields of vision, your eyes' adaptation to dark, and your color vision. He may also use the sophisticated electroretinogram, in which a contact lens that is connected to an electrode is placed on your cornea and instruments measure your retina's response to blinking lights.

You've probably heard and read lots about the marvelous new "space-age" treatments given with the *laser*, so we'll talk about that treatment first. "Laser" is a new word which began as an acronym for Light Amplification by Stimulated Emission of Radiation. It is a way of using electronics to create a perfectly parallel beam of light of one pure color. The beam can be controlled to thousandths of a millimeter widths and can be aimed through the cornea and lens with no damage and without producing any feeling. You simply lie there with your eye open as the doctor aims the beam at specific targets on the retina.

Laser treatment has been shown to be effective in early cases of diabetic retinopathy. The laser is focused on tiny bleeding arteries or veins to essentially heat-seal them. Used similarly, laser treatment has been used to save the eyes of infants with early stages of retrolental fibroplasia.

Actually, light was first used in the 1950s to "spotweld" retinal detachments with a device developed in Germany which produced an intense beam of brilliant conventional light from a xenon arc. This is called *photocoagulation*. When the laser came along in the 1960s, it was tried. Its lack of heat and its fine beam make it more precise, although some ophthalmologists still prefer the xenon arc device. With either instrument, the light is used to irritate the choroid under the retina so that it will form pinpoints of scar tissue that grab the retina from behind.

If the light treatment works, the scalpel can be spared. But it doesn't always work in simple cases of retinal detachment and seldom works in giant tears. Then the eye has to be operated on. First, the retinal edges must be coaxed back into their proper position. In the case of giant tears which fold over themselves like crinkled wallpaper, the unfolding is a difficult problem. One solution produced at the Retina Foundation in Boston is a special motor-driven operating table onto which you are strapped and which then rotates you into various positions to let gravity help unfold the retinal tear.

In any case, the idea is to get the retina to lie back on the choroid. Then the outside of the eye is irritated at specific points so that the choroid will produce scar tissue. This means the conjunctiva has to be opened, and perhaps a muscle cut so that the area of the retinal tear can be exposed. Then the doctor applies one of two kinds of irritants. The most common, and the one in longest use, is *surgical diathermy*. Here a needle carrying high-frequency electrical current is merely touched to points on the sclera. The resultant heat produces pinpoints of irritation and stimulates scar formation. A newer way to do this is with the supercold of a *cryoprobe*. In both cases, a hypodermic needle is inserted through the sclera just where the retina is detached, to draw out blood, vitreous, or any other fluids which have accumulated under the retina. Then the muscle is reattached exactly as it was, and the conjunctiva is closed.

Another kind of operation which is being used more and more is the *scleral buckle*. Here a thin channel is cut in the sclera just at the area where the retina is loose, and a tube of silicone rubber is pushed in and anchored. The idea is to literally buckle the sclera inward until it moves against the retina from behind.

There are three other, less widely-used ways to reattach retinas. One is the injection of vitreous humor directly into the eye to temporarily increase the internal pressure so as to push the retina back into place. The new vitreous humor is either taken from a donor eye or made of a new compound that closely resembles human vitreous humor. Of course, this procedure cannot be used if the eye already has glaucoma.

Another exotic treatment is the insertion into the eye of a needle which has a rubber balloon at its tip. Once in the eye, the balloon is inflated and used to push the retina back into place. It works especially well to help unfold the retina in giant tears. Equally exotic is a supersmall pair of scissors that is inserted into the eye to treat complicated cases where the retina is attached by tiny strands of scar tissue to the membrane that contains the vitreous. The scissors delicately cut these strands to free the retina, while not damaging the retina itself.

Retinal surgery, only half a century old, is now about eighty percent successful. If you are an older person with long-standing diabetes, you can expect to go back for laser treatments every few years to keep the bleeding under control. If your retina has been reattached, you may have some new blind spots that you will have to learn to live with. This depends largely on how long your retina was loose before it was treated by the doctor.

If you've had heat or cold treatments, you have to lie in bed, and quietly, for a month or month-and-a-half to allow those spotwelds to take—that is, to form firm scar tissue connections. Then you'll wear pinhole glasses to restrict your eye movements. Laser spotwelding treatments can be done on an outpatient basis, if the tear is small—incredible as that may seem.

If the cause of the bleeding or detachment of your retina is a cyst, the laser can often be used to successfully remove it. However, if the cause is a tumor pressing from behind, more extensive surgery most likely will be necessary. Tumors are the subject of the next chapter.

8. Tumor Operations

We don't like to think about it, but tissue in any part of the human body can begin growing in an unusual way. Such overgrowths of tissue usually are referred to as tumors. Doctors often call such new growths by the Greek term, *neoplasm*.

A tumor which grows slowly to a certain size and remains that size, and which is similar to surrounding tissue is usually referred to as a *benign* tumor. Warts and fatty tumors are examples. A tumor's benignancy refers to the fact that it will not spread. But even a benign tumor can cause trouble in an eye, by pressing on a nerve, or a blood vessel, or some other sensitive structure.

When a tumor is rapid and virulent in its growth, and differs from surrounding tissue, it is called *malignant*. A malignant tumor is, in a plain word, cancer. It grows uncontrollably; as it spreads it captures healthy tissue and converts it to its own diseased form. Cancers also send seed cells out through the lymph and blood systems. These seed cells may migrate to brain, lung, or other tissue, and set up satellite cancers—called *metastases*—there.

Eye cancers are doubly dangerous: they not only threaten vision, but life itself, especially since they are so close to the brain. Fortunately for most people, the eye is one of the least common of cancer sites. However, it is also true that cancers are known to develop in all structures of the eye.

Cancer, no matter where its site or what its form, is most readily curable when it is found in its original location and is treated early, while it is "young." Many cancers of the eye are quite visible and therefore reveal themselves quite early. Too often, however, the victim ignores the early warning signs and seeks out a doctor only when the cancer becomes unsightly, causes pain, or impairs vision. By then the cancer is quite advanced.

Today's doctor has an arsenal of weapons effective against tumors, including the scalpel, electric cautery, X-rays and other forms of radiation, and chemicals. All of these powerful agents are judiciously applied so as to be more destructive of tumor tissue than of surrounding healthy tissue. Again, while there are effective tumor treatments, all are most effective when applied early.

Our fear of blindness is second only to our fear of cancer. And when a person suspects he or she has a cancer that can cause blindness, the fear is multiplied. Sometimes people jump to conclusions and suspect blinding cancer without ever consulting a doctor. Self-diagnosis sometimes can be as dangerous as no diagnosis. Not every bump or red spot or pain in the eye is a sign of cancer. Actually, eye tumors can be accurately identified by the eye doctor only after careful examination of your eye, testing of its vision, and special laboratory tests.

There are, for instance, false tumors, or pseudotumors, which often fool even experts. These are masses which form for various reasons, and on first glance appear to be tumors. Years ago, before today's sophisticated diagnostic tests, many eyes were operated on, and even removed, in the belief that such eyes were cancerous. Such errors seldom occur today, thanks to the precision of examination of tissues under the microscope.

Many of these pseudotumors push the eye from behind so that it bulges forward. Doctors call this *exophthalmos*. It is also a frequent sign of thyroid disease, particularly hyperthyroidism, when it often occurs in both eyes. In any case, the doctor will check the health of your thyroid gland with radioiodine tracers and other tests if your eyes bulge. A tumor behind the eye also may reveal its presence by disturbances in vision. For instance, a famous golf pro was embarrassed at the tee when his wood refused to connect with the golf ball. He went to his family doctor who told him he had thyroid problems, and prescribed iodine medicine. But the visual problems continued. His left eye continued bulging badly and he soon had trouble closing the lids. He then consulted an ophthalmologist (RAP), and was sent to the X-ray department where some special radiopaque dye was injected into a vein on his forehead and X-ray pictures of his head were made. They revealed evidence of a tumor behind the left eye. He was operated on and the tumor was found and removed. The pathology laboratory reported it to be a *pseudolymphoma* that was neatly encapsulated, which meant that no other structures were involved. After a few weeks, the pro was back on the links, his vision restored.

Probably the most common pseudotumor is *granuloma*, a bumpy-surfaced growth. Other kinds of nontumorous lumps which can form behind and around the eye, and even in the eye, include cysts, accumulations of fat (*xanthomas* and *lipomas*), and blood vessel bumps called *hemangiomas*. Pouches of bacterial infection can also cause serious pressures on the eye, especially when caused by tuberculosis, syphilis, and tularemia bacteria.

More tumors occur around the eye than in the eye. These are usually removed with chemicals and with techniques of plastic surgery which we'll describe in the next chapter. The lower lid and the inner corner of the eye are the most usual sites of such tumors, especially of skin cancers known as *epitheliomas* (which can occur anywhere on the face). These cancers occur most frequently in people fifty to fifty-five years of age, and slightly more frequently in men than in women. Irritation and exposure to sunlight are two factors which may help produce such growths. Epitheliomas also develop on the conjunctiva and on the cornea, although rarely.

The most common tumors in eyes are distinguished by a color ranging from tan to black. Since color pigment is technically called *melanin*, these tumors are usually called *melanomas*. Melanomas grow slowly in those structures of the eye which are pigmented. The most obvious location is the iris, which has a greater or lesser amount of pigment, on which its color depends (blue, hazel, brown, etc.), as we explained in Chapter 2. No iris is perfectly uniform in color. Because it is made of muscle fibers which radiate from the pupil, it has lines of color arranged like the rays of the sun. It also has areas of more and less color. In fact, each iris is a unique design of nature's artful use of color. Like snow-flakes, no two irises are alike.

Some irises have "freckles," flecks of light or dark brown color. Freckles are usually harmless deposits of pigment. But when flecks grow or when the freckled part of the iris opens or closes a bit sluggishly, the fleck may be of a more serious nature; it may be a melanoma.

The eye doctor is suspicious of every fleck. He will look carefully at it with a special kind of microscope called a *gonioscope* (also used in glaucoma, see Chapter 5). He will search for the tiny blood vessels which feed such tumors, and he will measure the angle the iris makes with the cornea. Usually a special contact lens is placed on the cornea to give the gonioscope the optics necessary to see into that iris-corneal corner.

Thanks to the development of surgery under the micro-scope, such tiny tumors can now be successfully cut out of the iris. The *iridectomy* technique is similar to that used to treat acute glaucoma. Minute attention is paid to leaving strands of muscle so that even with a segment missing, the iris, after it heals, can still function. Most importantly, the rest of the eye can be saved.

Melanomas are not always limited to a fleck but may extend into the ciliary body or into the choroid. If the dark fleck is an extension of a tumor in the ciliary body or the choroid, then the entire tumor must be treated. Where the tumor is located, and how extensive it is are two very important considerations. Your doctor has to know the answers to both questions before he can start treatment. Flecks on the iris can easily be seen, but tumors of the choroid are hidden. Microsurgery can often save the eye even when the melanoma extends into the ciliary body.

Sometimes the first hint of the presence of a melanoma is when some vision is lost in one eye; examination shows it to be a detached retina. As we explained in Chapter 7, eye surgeons will always suspect tumors of the choroid when they see through their ophthalmoscope a retina which has detached, even though very few retinas actually become detached because of tumors. The idea is this: if they suspect it, they can look for the tumor; not finding it, they can go on and treat the detachment for what it is, and that is serious enough.

Sometimes the pressure from the tumor not only detaches the retina, but also causes glaucoma, and even a cataract, which serve to complicate the situation, confuse attempts at diagnosis, and continually interfere with vision.

Tumors of the vitreous body and choroid are very difficult to diagnose before surgery. The doctor will look for clues such as enlarged, or an overabundant supply of, blood vessels in the area, and various other signs that can be seen by special kinds of illumination.

If your melanoma is limited to a freckle on the iris, consider yourself very lucky. Of course, the surgeon will not be absolutely sure it is so limited until the report comes back from the pathology laboratory. There, the cut-away tissue will be finely sliced and samples will be studied under a microscope. If the pathologist finds that all of the malignancy was confined to a speck and that there was only healthy tissue around it, that means that the entire tumor was removed. You should also know that melanomas may form at more than one location in the eye—although only very rarely.

One of the most vicious eye cancers is *retinoblastoma*, which typically occurs in young children, although every once in a while an adult develops it. Typical of the approximately one hundred children affected by this cancer in the United States every year, is a white child whose parents noticed the condition when the child was two years old. In about a third of the cases, both eyes are affected.

Although it has been extensively studied, retinoblastoma is a kind of cancer which is difficult to treat successfully. First noted by medical authorities in the year 1597, it is now known to occur in two forms. One form, which occurs in twenty percent of cases, seems to be inherited, although scientists haven't yet worked out the statistics or the mechanism of its inheritance. Persons who have a relative with retinoblastoma, and who carry its gene, have a ten to fifty percent chance of having a child with it. The other kind is not inherited.

Of course, it's all academic to the young victim. His parents first notice that something is wrong when they spot what is known as the "cat's-eye reflex." If you have a cat or have ever shined a flashlight or headlight into a cat's eyes, you'll know what this is. It is a bright reflection of white or pale yellow light which shines back at you from the pupil. Healthy children's eyes often reflect bright pink when light is flashed into them. In the last chapter we explained why photographs of children often depict them with "pink pinholes" at the center of their eyes. An eye with retinoblastoma shines instead with a white reflection in photographs taken with flashbulbs or electronic flash.

Retinoblastoma is vicious because it so readily invades the optic nerve. If you remember the facts about the retina which we detailed in Chapter 2, you can understand why. The nerve fibers (which carry the retina's image of what the eye is looking at) converge at the optic nerve. Therefore, retinoblastoma, which is a cancer that arises in the retina, follows nerve pathways as it grows. Once it takes over the optic nerve, there is little to stop it from invading the skull and there spreading its disease to the brain. At the same time, this dangerous growth also has a strong propensity to send seed cells into the blood stream and to spread its malignancy to other parts of the body in this way; in fact, some retinoblastoma seed cells start satellite cancers as far away as the liver, kidney, and testes, as well as close by in the head.

Unfortunately, because it strikes such very young children and because there are no clues that anything is wrong until the cat's-eye reflex is noticed, most retinoblastomas are well advanced by the time a doctor gets to see and diagnose it. The reflection in the pupil is from the pale surface of the cancer itself. The most telltale sign which the doctor sees with his ophthalmoscope is deposits of calcium on the diseased retina. These can also be seen in X-ray films of the eye.

Unlike melanomas, which seem to worsen with radiation, retinoblastomas are very susceptible to such treatment. Some doctors like to use the radioactive gas of radium (known as *radon*). Others prefer to use X-rays beamed with special equipment right into the eye. The main problem is that a dose of radiation strong enough to kill the cancer might also harm or destroy the delicate structures at the front of the eye, particularly the cornea and lens. Instead, the radiation has to be beamed into the side of the eye; at such an angle it may not be as effective.

Several cancers which originate outside the eye but invade it. Among the most invasive, quickest-growing, and dangerous are those which begin in the lid muscles. They are *sarcomas* with the long names of *rhabdomyoma, rhabdomyosarcoma, myosarcoma,* and *myoblastoma.* The worst of these villains is rhabdomyosarcoma which usually occurs in youngsters aged about six years. *Gliomas* are brain tumors which invade the eye via the optic nerve. And there are cancers of the bone and lymph around the eye which can also affect it.

The eye can also capture the seed cells of cancers located in distant parts of the body. These metastases are just as threatening to vision and life as are cancers which originate in the eye. A study at Montefiore Hospital and Medical Center, New York, showed that over a third of patients with breast cancer had metastases to the eye. Other research studies have indicated that seventy percent of metastatic cancers of eyes came from original cancer sites in the breast. Lung, cervical, and prostatic cancers are also frequent sites. Most metastases, no matter their origin, take root in the *uvea* (iris, ciliary body, choroid).

One of the most horrendous decisions an eye surgeon has to make is whether or not to remove an eye, and if so, when. This is particularly distressing to him when the eye is that of a young child, as is frequently the case. Often the decision fairly well makes itself, as the cancer has already destroyed vision and is threatening life. But sometimes there is some vision left. If the tumor seems benign, or if radiation seems to be helping, the surgeon may elect to stay his knife. However, if it is fast growing, he will want to remove the eye immediately, knowing that the eye cannot be saved and restored but can only bring further problems. Often the cancer can spread to the other, good, eye. But even more serious is the fact that it can spread to other parts of the body and even the brain, causing death.

These are words that strike fear in anyone's heart: cancer and death. But they unfortunately become the facts of life to some people—perhaps to you, or to someone close to you. If that is the case, you need to be advised that the best course is to listen to your doctor and have the eye removed. It's quite all right to go to another ophthalmologist for another diagnosis and a confirming opinion; in fact, your own family doctor may refer you to one; or, the first eye doctor may do so. But don't shop around, visiting a dozen doctors, or even quacks, in the vain hope that the cancer can be made to evaporate. It just won't happen. If it's an advanced melanoma, retinoblastoma, glioma or sarcoma, your life is in jeopardy while you are delaying your decision.

Actually, the removal of an eye is a safe and short operation, often done under local anesthesia. There are two ways to remove an eye: *evisceration* and *enucleation*. In evisceration, the contents of the eyeball—lens, iris, vitreous—are scooped out and a glass sphere is inserted. Later, a scleral contact lens may be placed over the eye so that it looks and moves normally. Evisceration is seldom done when there is a cancer present, since there is always the danger that some small spot of malignancy may remain, to spread later and threaten health and life. Instead, enucleation or total removal of the eyeball is performed.

Despite the emotional impact of such an operation, it is really quite safe. Essentially it begins like most eye operations, with the conjunctiva cut at the limbus—where the white meets the clear (or once clear) cornea. The conjunctiva is then stretched open, and the anesthetized eye is cut free from Tenon's capsule and the six muscles attached to it. The surgeon severs the optic nerve and cauterizes the cut retinal blood vessels to stop bleeding. He works slowly—sometimes with a scalpel, sometimes with a wire loop called a snare—so as to limit bleeding. Then muscles and membrane are tied together, the conjunctiva sewn closed, and the eye is covered with bandages.

The removed, cancerous eye is sent to the laboratory for detailed analysis under the microscope. This is not only to pinpoint the diagnosis, but to assure the surgeon that he has taken out all of the tumor.

A glass sphere is placed in the empty *orbit*, or eyesocket, and the muscles and Tenon's capsule are attached to it so that it will move in concert with its real mate. Then the conjunctiva is closed at the front and covered with a realistic, plastic cornea.

Glass and plastic eyes today are tailored so closely to the remaining eye that they defy detection by all but eye surgeons, and then only on close examination.

Once you or your loved one has recovered and is active again, the life that was saved will be sweet indeed. There will be not even a hint to the outside world that it is being seen through only one real eye.

9. Plastic Surgery

Most people think of plastic surgery as a means of making them better-looking. That is only partly true. It is actually a branch of surgery with its own techniques for removing and repairing tissue of, or just under, the skin, usually on or around the face. In many cases, such as straightening a hooked nose, all of the tissue which is removed is healthy. In other cases, such as the removal of a skin tumor, much of the tissue involved is diseased.

Plastic surgery is no longer rare. About 100,000 plastic surgery procedures of the eyes alone are performed every year in the United States. While most involve the eyelids, some are performed on the areas immediately around the eye, such as the brows.

Most of this chapter will be devoted to detailing the common eye conditions needing plastic surgery, one of which will apply to you. But first you should understand some philosophy and other general considerations of plastic surgery if you or a loved one is going to undergo such an eye operation.

To begin with, plastic surgery is not new. Records from ancient Egypt and India show that surgery to improve appearance was attempted thousands of years ago. In fact, plastic surgery was probably the first form of surgery. Today's plastic surgery, largely the refinement of techniques developed to restore men disfigured in World Wars I and II, has been called "surgery of millimeters," because that is the narrow margin between pleasing and poor cosmetic results. These are important millimeters. Each millimeter can have a mile of emotional repercussion. This is especially true for eyes, which can look hideous or beautiful with a millimeter one way or another.

Because they are aware of the heavy psychological impact of such operations, surgeons frequently spend as much time sitting down and talking to patients as in operating on them. They keep alert for the mentally disturbed patient, especially the paranoid who fantasizes that other people are making fun of essentially normal looks. Many of these kinds of patients travel from surgeon to surgeon. Some manage to have several cosmetic operations over the years when what they really need is psychiatric help, not surgery.

Weeding out such disturbed people is just one reason surgeons talk at length to prospective cosmetic patients. During the interview, the surgeon will try to evaluate just what the emotionally stable person wants from surgery. And the doctor will explain that improvement, not perfection, is the best that can be achieved. "Plastic surgery," says the American Academy of Facial Plastic and Reconstructive Surgery, "will not serve as a cure-all for the individual who blames his appearance for lack of success in life."

People who turn to plastic surgery should learn what is in store for them, in terms of discomfort, rehabilitation, and expense. Plastic surgery does not produce instant results. It can make wonderful changes in looks, but it cannot make these changes suddenly. Surgeons, after all, are skilled men, not magicians. And no matter how minor the procedure, liv-

ing tissue is being cut, bruised, shoved, and shaped, in the
process. Such disruptions can lead to temporary pain, swelling, and discoloration. While all of these disappear as healing
progresses, they still must be suffered.

Although healing takes weeks, even months, most people
who have had cosmetic eye surgery are up and around again
in a day. This usually means you can soon go back to school
or to work or to housekeeping. Although there is usually
some discomfort during the first days after surgery, it is not
at all unbearable and it soon leaves.

Any operation, plastic or otherwise, leaves scars. Scars are
inevitable whenever skin is cut. But the eye surgeon knows
how to hide them. Skin folds are places where a neat scar
can be naturally hidden. Conscious as they are of millimeters,
eye surgeons are extremely careful about realigning cut skin
ends and are meticulous in their suturing, placing most
stitches under the surface and operating with the help of a
magnifying lens or microscope. In fact, they make most fine
seamstresses look like amateurs.

You should also realize that healing progresses in phases.
Wounds look fairly good when the stitches come out. In the
next phase, the young scars get to looking awful. They
become red, thick, raised, tender, and even lumpy. This lasts
for about three months, during which you may be tempted
to tell your eye doctor to redo it. Just about then, however,
the scar starts to shrink into a thin line that is barely visible,
the lumpiness disappears, and the area is no longer as sensitive to heat and cold. When the redness fades completely,
you may have to look hard in the mirror to find any scar
at all. This entire process takes about six months, so don't
be impatient.

One other consideration: plastic surgery in real life is not
like plastic surgery in the movies. There, as the heroine's
bandages are breathlessly removed, an incredibly beautiful
face is revealed. Actually, when your bandages are removed,
you'll see eyes that are somewhat puffy and somewhat red-

dened. Like most good things of life, postsurgical beauty takes time to acquire, and a full six months of healing.

Eye operations that involve plastic surgery are performed in that small area from the eyebrow to the cheekbone, and mostly on the upper and lower lids.

BAGGY EYELIDS (called *blepharochalasis* or *dermatochalasis of the eyelid*) is perhaps the most common eye condition treated by plastic surgery. Baggy lids seem to be a result of aging, since they occur most frequently after age fifty. While both sexes suffer equally often from this condition, more men than women seek to have their baggy lids lifted by surgery. Often the operation is solely for cosmetic reasons, but in many instances, especially when the upper lids sag, it is necessary to restore vision. Many people with baggy upper eyelids have to tilt their heads back in order to see under the fold of the drooping flesh. (This is somewhat the same technique which people with *ptosis*, or droopy lids, use to see; see below.)

There are two kinds of baggy eyelids. In the simpler kind, the skin sags as the result of having lost its elasticity. This comes as a consequence of aging, as skin tissue, like a rubber band, loses its springiness, or its bounce. In the less simple kind, fat has pushed through from the eye socket below in a process known as *orbital herniation*. When this happens, the eyelid not only sags, but puffs out as well.

To correct simple baggy eyelids, the surgeon in essence grabs a pinch of eyelid skin and pulls it until it is taut. Then he cuts away that excess skin and sews the remaining edges together. Of course, he does this with extreme care and precision. He'll be sure that the incision line in the upper lid is made exactly where the lid skin has a natural fold. If the brow droops, too, there will be one at the brow line. The incision line of the lower lid will most likely be just below the edge of the lid so the lashes can hide it.

To correct the more serious kind of baggy lid, the surgeon must cut down to the eyeball socket edge. He may do this

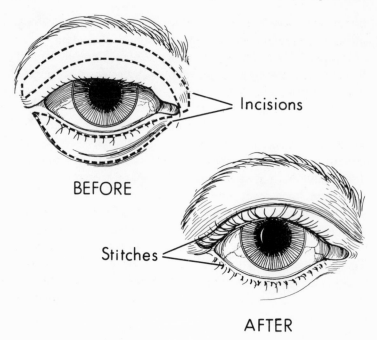

FIG. 10. Blepharoplasty. Plastic surgery to correct baggy eyelids involves cutting out a pinch of loose flesh and sewing the cut ends together. Cutting and sewing are done at natural lines so as to be invisible after healing.

first by puncturing the "bag" at the outer corner of the eye and letting the pressure push the accumulated fat out. Then he will insert an instrument to scrape away any remaining fat. Sometimes, when the fat deposits have been removed, the bagginess disappears. Usually, however, it remains and some sagging skin has to be pinched and cut away as in the simpler form of baggy lids.

In any case, the tissue behind the lids has to be sealed to prevent more fat from pushing forward. Cautery, a form of electrical heat, can do this through the small hole in the skin at the edge of the eye. Some surgeons, however, prefer to open up the eyelid, remove the fat, and suture the opening in the eyesocket tissue through which the fat has seeped.

Either way can be effective, depending on which technique the surgeon prefers and the situation calls for.

Usually both the upper and lower lids are operated on, but this is not always necessary. Again, it depends on your situation. The operation for both lids takes three to four hours.

RELAXED LIDS result in either the turning in or the turning out of the edge, or margin. When a lid—usually the lower lid—turns out it is called *ectropion*. This can be dangerous, since it allows the tears to spill out, leaving the eye dry. Many older people who are constantly wiping spilled tears from their eyes suffer ectropion. If the eye becomes dry, irritation (conjunctivitis), drying of the cornea, and possibly infection can follow.

When the edge of the eyelid turns in, it is called *entropion*. This can happen to both the upper and lower lids and when it does so, the eyelashes will rub against the eye, irritating it and possibly scratching the cornea. Untreated, infection and blindness can follow.

Both *ectropion* and *entropion* can be corrected by relatively simple and short plastic operations, in which wedges or slices of tissue are taken from the eyelid to permanently reposition it and make it taut.

SLANTED EYES, or *epicanthus*, is not a disease, but inherited anatomy. It is typical among the Oriental races classified as Mongoloids (especially Chinese and Japanese). It is actually a web of overhanging tissue that is part of the upper lid at the corner near the nose. Some scientists think it is a remnant of the nictating membrane which other animals, besides man, have—in the same way that the appendix is an evolutionary remnant. The nictating membrane is a third lid in animals. You've probably seen it: As your dog is about to fall asleep and his outer lids are closing, the red nictating membrane slides over the eyeball. The eyeballs of Orientals are globe-shaped, as are those of Occidentals, but the eye opening is made oblong by the epicanthus.

Oriental eyes can become "round eyes" with a simple

operation in which the epicanthus is cut and, in effect, opened until that corner of the upper lid is freed of its attachment. The shape of the incision—called Z-plasties by surgeons—opens the tissue without leaving noticeable scars.

DROOPY LIDS are known medically as *ptosis* (the "p" is silent). There are two kinds. One kind is congenital. It runs in some families so that some of the children in a family will be born with droopy eyes. Sometimes the ptosis is one of a group of malformations a child is born with, including small cornea, and missing segment of the iris. When that combination occurs, it means there was some error of development before birth as the uvea* of the eye was being formed.

Ptosis can also be acquired by older children or adults. Then, the cause is usually faulty control of the *levator* muscle. A common cause in adults is stroke, as control centers in the brain are crippled or destroyed by hemorrhage or blood starvation. Muscular diseases, such as *myasthenia gravis*, also make themselves known by causing ptosis.

Droopy upper lids are considered "sexy" by some people, as is reflected in the term sometimes used for the condition: "bedroom eyes." But, as we noted above for baggy eyes, the person suffering the condition has to tilt his head back severely in order to see from under those sagging lids. Normally, the upper lid follows rather perfectly so that the line of the lid "floats" on the top of the black dot that is the pupil, that opening formed by the iris. If the lid line is *in* the pupil, then it is blocking out the top part of the picture the eye sees, much as if you put your hand over part of the lens of your camera.

Plastic surgery can correct both congenital and acquired ptosis. Usually the eyelid is cut open so that the levator muscle (the muscle which raises the lid) is exposed. Then a segment of it is trimmed away from the bottom and the muscle

---

*Uvea includes iris, ciliary body, and choroid.

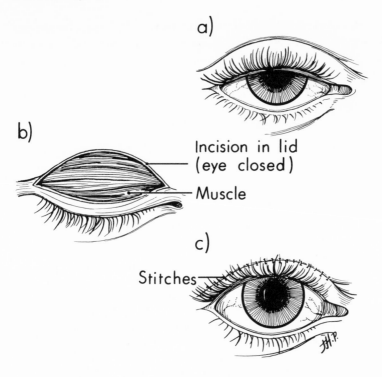

a)

b)

Incision in lid
(eye closed)

Muscle

c)

Stitches

FIG. 11. **Ptosis.** Droopy eyelid is corrected by an operation in which a section of muscle is cut out. Sewn back, the eyelid muscle pulls tighter, lifting the lid to its normal position on top of the pupil.

is reattached to the *tarsus*, that part of the eyelid which is made of cartilage. In the case of children born with ptosis, the correcting operation is usually recommended at ages four to six, when they can tolerate general anesthesia and before they develop permanent neck problems. Because both eyes are affected, both of the child's eyes will be operated on, although sometimes only one is done at each operation.

In adults with acquired ptosis, one eye alone often droops; in that case, only the affected eye needs the operation, obviously. In rare cases where the levator muscle is paralyzed, other muscles can be brought in to do the job of lifting the eyelid. One is the *frontalis* muscle of the forehead. Another is the *superior rectus* muscle of the eyeball: as the eye is lifted, so is the upper lid.

SPOTS, CYSTS, INFECTIONS, and GROWTHS of the eyelids and around the eye are very common and can be successfully removed surgically. The most common spots have the difficult name of *xanthelasma*, also known as *palpebral xanthelasma*. These are flat, smooth yellowish growths usually found on the lids near the corner of the eye over the nose. More women than men seem to have these apparently harmless deposits of fat, which also are closely associated with high blood cholesterol. Sometimes reducing the amount of saturated fats (eggs, butter, cream) in the diet can make an xanthelasma wither. However, the surest way to remove one is by surgery.

Cysts of the eyelid are common. Called *chalazion* by doctors, they develop when sebaceous (oil) glands of the lid are blocked; then infection sets in. The result is a tiny pealike and painful mass of liquid in the lid. Sometimes hot compresses help to open the cyst, but more usually the surgeon has to pull the lid back and quickly cut the cyst away under a local anesthetic. He does not even have to stitch the cut closed; it heals itself unseen. An eye patch will have to be worn for only a day.

A sty (*hordeolum*) is an infection of the base of the eyelash, and especially of a gland of Zeis or Moll located there (and from which the sty gets its formal name). Children often have sties as a result of wiping their eyes with dirty fingertips. Often the whitish pus and redness go away when hot compresses and antibiotics are applied. But more stubborn infections have to be cut by the surgeon, and the infection squeezed out. Antibiotic ointments applied for several days help prevent any residual infection from spreading. No scar remains.

Tumors, mostly benign but some malignant, seem to have

an affinity for eyes, and many of them require immediate surgery. Moles or freckles around the eye and especially the eyelids have to be watched constantly, particularly if you are past fifty years of age. There is always the chance that a spot of color will become malignant and develop into a *melanoma*. Cauliflowerlike growths which sometimes look like giant warts and are called *papillomas* prefer lid margins. These unsightly but harmless growths can be easily removed by merely surgically slicing them off of the surface, since they do not have "roots," as cancers do.

The most common cancer of the eyelid is *basal cell carcinoma* or *epithelioma* which usually occurs on the lid margin and often is confused with an open sore. *Squamous cell* skin cancers, a related kind, are less frequent and usually reveal themselves as whiter or more glistening. Less often seen by eye surgeons are such skin cancers as *adenoepithelioma, trichoepithelioma*, and *syringoma* which start in lid glands, hair follicles, or sweat glands, respectively.

Sometimes X-ray or other radiation treatment can be used as part of the treatment of an eyelid cancer. Especially if it is a large one, the radiation can help shrink it to a more manageable size. Almost always, the cancer has to be excised, or cut out. Eyelid cancers are often the severest test of the eye surgeon's plastic skills. First, he has to be sure that he removes all of the cancerous tissue, plus a small margin of healthy tissue around it. Then, he has to repair the damage in such a way that the eyelid will function properly and look as though little, if anything, has been removed. Often large segments of an eyelid can be removed without the casual observer, months later, noticing it. The occurrence of most growths at the edge or margin of the eyelid helps. Also helpful is that these growths usually occur in mature people whose skin has a lot of sag. In fact, in most instances, patients look younger after having a lid cancer removed than before!

As we said early in the chapter, the healing process is

long, so don't expect instant beauty. Instead, take good care of your eyes. Bandages can usually come off in twenty-four hours, after which you *must* keep the wound scrupulously clean. Your doctor may instruct you to keep ice packs on it to reduce swelling and to wash it with peroxide or warm water and to follow that with a gentle massage with hydrocortisone ointment to hasten healing (knead the closed eye with the fingertips, but do it gently). Stitches usually can come out in the doctor's office five or six days after your plastic surgery. There is no pain.

10. Before and After Your Eye Operation

As we said at the beginning of this book, the decision to have an eye operation should mean the beginning of treatment that will return your sight to normal, or certainly vastly improve it. It is a decision which should be reached jointly by you and your eye doctor, and preferably with the consultation and concurrence of your own family doctor. Thus, it should be a three-way decision: the surgeon knows the eye condition and the surgical chances for its successful correction; your family doctor knows the state of your health and your ability to physically and psychologically bear the surgery, and you know best how you feel about taking the risk (no matter how small), and about your ability to pay for the operation and hospitalization.

If surgery is the best answer to your eye problem, it is also the most drastic—and the most dramatic. As safe as modern surgery and modern anesthesia are, they are still not without danger. No surgery is 100 percent effective in its curative powers, although eye operations are among the most successful, as you can see by this table:

Operation	Rate of Success (in percent)
Muscle imbalance correction	90
Corneal transplants:	
cone cornea	90
degenerative diseases	50
cornea destroyed by acids or alkali	5
Glaucoma:	
acute	95
chronic	70
Cataract removal	90
(Microsurgical technique)	95
Retinal detachments	60
Tumor operations	depends on kind of tumor and extent of its growth
Plastic surgery	90

Various factors can keep an operation from being perfectly successful. The anatomy of your eye may be abnormal so that the surgeon cannot perfectly complete the operation the way he usually does. Or, the problem may be more extensive or more deteriorated than the surgeon originally diagnosed and expected. Sometimes, the problem is complicated by other factors. Infection can creep in and delay the tissues' healing.

When such complications arise, and the success of the operation is not complete, another, second, operation may be necessary. When performed, it may lead to total success, but that does not always happen.

Just remember, the surgeon is as interested in achieving such total success as you are. True, it's your eye and your sight that are at stake, so you have more to risk. But his professional reputation and his future referrals are also at stake. Remember, too, that surgeons are often driven people who are success-oriented, and who hate to fail.

Sometimes second operations are necessary because the patient doesn't heed the surgeon's advice. For instance, of the twenty-five percent of retinas which are repaired, then become detached again, almost all occur in people who ignore or forget advice to avoid sudden jerks, blows to the head, contact sports, straining and lifting of heavy objects.

You may get impatient and start nagging your physician about letting you have an operation to restore your sight. Don't be so certain that surgery is the magic answer. And don't be so certain that it is all that easy. Taken as a whole, a surgical operation represents a certain degree of stress on your eye and your body. What your doctor has to weigh is whether the stress is worth it. Unless it is an emergency situation, he's apt to be conservative and say, ''Let's wait a while longer.''

Of course, the opposite might be true in your case. It may develop that your doctor has decided that an operation would be best for you and it is *you* who are delaying it. If so, remember that every day you delay having your operation is another unnecessary day of poor vision. If your own doctor recommends it and the surgeon has examined you, studied your case, and agrees, and the operation will take place in a legitimate hospital, you should go through with it. You know your doctor and trust him (or he would not be your doctor). You probably don't know the eye surgeon, but if your doctor recommends him you should accept his recommendation.

What's more, every operation that a surgeon performs is reviewed in microscopic detail by committees of fellow doctors on the staff of the hospital. One, for instance, is the Tissue Committee, which examines every bit of tissue cut by surgeons at that hospital. A surgeon has to be able to prove that the operations he performs are absolutely necessary, or he stands to lose his privileges of using the hospital's operating room. Governmental agencies and insurance companies which help pay for hospitalization and surgery are also interested and keep close tabs on what is occurring in operating rooms.

Being afraid of the hospital and the operation is quite natural. But you can stem your fears with information. That, in fact, is one reason for this book. A publication* of the American College of Surgeons put it well:

> In studies of the emotional responses of hospital patients, psychologists have found that the fears patients have, except in the most critical cases, are not fear of pain, or disability, or death, but simply apprehension and anxiety about the unknown. To the outsider, hospital people and hospital procedures are mysterious, and too often, nobody takes time to tell the fearful patient what is going on, and why. As a result, his imagination builds threats of things that never happen. He envisions risks that don't exist. Surprisingly, these irrational fears may be found among hospital patients of all educational, social and economic backgrounds.

Just remember that surgery has never been as safe—and as effective—as it is today. Your surgeon will be working with the aid of magnifying lenses or an operating microscope to make the smallest incisions and do the most accurate rejoining of tissues that is humanly possible. Consider this: he'll be using micro-point needles that are a third of a millimeter in diameter (0.013 inch) or less; these needles pull sutures that are only as thick as three side-by-side red blood cells (size 10-0 sutures are 22 microns of .0009 inch thick!).

A.C.S. Bulletin, January 1973.

BEFORE YOUR OPERATION

You will be thoroughly examined by the surgeon, even though your own physician has carefully examined you. The surgeon will go over any X-rays and laboratory test results so that he knows everything about your eye that he can. He will also order tests to evaluate the state of health of your heart and lungs, the condition of your blood, and will search for hidden conditions such as diabetes and kidney disease, which either require special consideration in surgery or which may (if severe enough) make surgery too dangerous.

He will spend a lot of time asking you about yourself and any previous operations you've had, even dental operations. For instance, the doctor will want to know if you've ever had trouble after a tooth was pulled, especially if the gum took a very long time to stop bleeding. He will also ask if you are allergic to any foods, or to any drugs such a penicillin. He will want to know if you are taking any medicine regularly—if so, which, when, and how much.

You will probably be asked to report to the hospital for admission the afternoon or night before your surgery is scheduled. In most hospitals, the operating room schedule starts very early in the morning, so your doctor will want you all ready for your operation as soon as you are awakened in the morning. This means that after you are admitted you will be shown to your room, where you can undress and go to bed. The doctor or a hospital representative should have told you to bring only necessary items, and none of any monetary value. When you go to the hospital for your operation, be sure to bring with you only the essentials:

> —No more than $5 in cash to pay for magazines, newspapers, etc., for the time you will feel well enough to thumb through them.
> —Travel clock
> —Small radio

—Personal-sized television (if allowed)
—Toiletries such as toothbrush, toothpaste, comb, brush, shaving or cosmetic items
—Pajamas (two pairs), robe, and slippers
—Nothing of value. Hospitals are public places, where such things are often lost or stolen.

In some hospitals, you fill out preadmission forms at home, then mail them in. If not, bring your Blue Cross-Blue Shield card or identification of other hospitalization-major medical insurance plan, or else bring a check to pay the hospital for its care. Operations are expensive. But you have to remember that the hospital (unless it is one of the few remaining *proprietary* hospitals) is a nonprofit community hospital. It therefore cannot and does not make any money. In fact, it loses money, and that's why it has to ask for public donations every year to remain open.

Once you are settled down, more routine tests will be made, such as blood and urine analyses. You'll be given an enema. If you seem the least bit anxious, the nurse will give you some tranquilizer or a sedative to calm and quiet you. You may also be given extra large doses of regular vitamins such as A, C, D, and various B's, as well as unusual ones such as K (to help your blood clot in a more efficient manner). You may be allowed a snack before bedtime.

In the morning, you will be awakened about 6 a.m., and fed a very light breakfast, such as toast and tea or decaffeinated coffee. You'll be medicated further with *Demerol*, a synthetic morphine, to put you in a state of near-sleep, and *Thorazine* to prevent nausea. Your face will be thoroughly washed with medicated soap and your eyelashes trimmed all the way down (they'll grow back in about six weeks). If your eye looks "beefy" or irritated, tiny samples of your conjunctiva will be painlessly scraped by an ophthalmology resident who will send this to the lab for drug sensitivity testing. Then he'll place an antibiotic ointment under your eyelids to keep any germs away. Special eye medicines may be given, to dilate your pupil, to lower the intraocular pressure, or whatever—depending on the operation you're scheduled for.

Your head (you should have been instructed to shower and shampoo before coming to the hospital) will be covered with a cap to contain your hair. Eyebrows are seldom shaved, but covered during surgery.

YOUR OPERATION

When your operating time is near, you will be transferred from your bed to a cart and wheeled to a holding area just outside the operating room. You'll be doing a lot of ceiling gazing at this stage, and you'll also be drowsy, so the hushed voices and the gowned doctors and nurses that speed by as you wait will be but a blur.

Finally, you'll be wheeled into the operating room. Unless you've seen one before (and even if you have) it will seem a bewildering place with a big operating light over trays of gleaming instruments. A two-eyed microscope covered with a plastic sheet will stand nearby. The nurses and your surgeon will be gowned and masked as at some ritual.

Indeed, the ritual begins with you being lifted off the cart and onto the operating table. Chances are, you'll be awake during the entire operation. This is because most ophthalmologists prefer for technical reasons (involving control and side-effects) to operate with their patients under local anesthesia, rather than under gas, or general anesthesia. Already heavily medicated, you will be in a light sleeplike state in which you'll be dozing most of the time, yet aware that there is activity around you. You'll be able to respond when your name is gently called, and far in the distance you'll hear the murmur of the surgeons' voices.

Once you are on the table, anesthetic will be dropped into

your eye. Your eyelids will be scrubbed with green soap and water. Then local anesthetic (sometimes mixed with epinephrine to lengthen its pain-killing effects) will be injected around the eye, in the brow, cheeks, and at the ear, in order to deaden certain facial nerves at their roots. Once the areas around the eye are deadened of pain, the surgeon will inject the anesthetic into the socket and behind the eye (*retrobulbar injection*). This is to temporarily paralyze the muscles of the eye. After this injection, the surgeon may gently massage the eyeball so as to help the medicine diffuse behind the eyeball. Then he'll ask you (you can respond to inquiries and commands, remember) to look up, down, right and left. If the anesthesia has taken its effect, the eye will be immobile, as well as free of feeling. Then the surgeon will clamp the eyelids open, run a curved needle around the eye muscle and turn it the way he needs to for the operation. Next, he'll position his microscope over the eye, and start to work with his tiny scalpel, and tinier needles and sutures. Always, he or his assistant are dropping sterile saline solution onto the conjunctiva to keep it moist.

If your doctor feels he can best operate while you are under general anesthesia (as for a child or for a cancer operation), he will be helped by an anesthesiologist, a physician you may never see (or the anesthetist, who is a specially trained nurse). He or she gives the "gas," which, when you inhale it, puts you into a sort of semisleep from which you can answer if called, but otherwise you are not aware of either your body or your surroundings. Or you may get a combination of local anesthetic and gas. The anesthesia has to be carefully selected because there are special considerations in eye surgery. You have to be maintained on a plane of anesthesia that allows you to breath regularly and lightly, so that your breathing will not make your diaphragm oscillate too heavily and jar your eye.

While you are asleep, the anesthesiologist will insert a

breathing tube into your mouth. Called an endotracheal tube, its purposes are to keep your airway open and to prevent your aspirating, or breathing in, any contents of your stomach that may be vomited as a sudden reaction.

AFTER YOUR SURGERY

If you've had gas, you will "come to" and regain consciousness in the recovery room, a special room with oxygen, all kinds of instruments, and lots of nurses to care for your special postoperative needs. You'll be there for several hours as nurses watch you and help you to emerge from the anesthesia. They'll call your name and squeeze your hand and make sure you respond and start trying to wake up. This is for your own good. You won't hurt, but your natural reflexes will return with consciousness.

Back in your room and somewhat aware of your surroundings again, you'll notice that you are very thirsty. This is partly because of fluids lost in surgery and partly because of the fact that the anesthetic gases were so dry.

If you've been operated on with only local injections of anesthesia, chances are you'll be returned right to your room. This is another reason eye surgeons prefer local to general anesthesia. Back in your room, in either case, you will be allowed to drink fluids to quench your thirst, but be given no solid foods (lest you develop nausea). The day after surgery you'll be allowed to eat a bland soft diet, such as eggs and cottage cheese, along with vitamin pills. On the third day you'll be back on solid foods again.

During these days after surgery, you'll be given enough codeine and other pain-killing pills to be comfortable. You'll also be given plenty of vitamins, and when the doctor changes the bandages over your eye he will be sure to place prednisolone ointment in it to hold down irritation, and antibiotic ointment to hold off bacterial infections. Other than that, there will not be much to do. You can have visitors if they will talk pleasantly and not worry or upset you. And you can listen as much as you like to your radio.

Lying there in your bed, you are, of course, excitedly curious about your vision. You probably can't wait to have the bandages removed so you can tell if your vision has been restored; at the same time you are just a bit fearful to find out. Could you be one of the small percentage of failures? You need to have a very positive attitude. After all, the odds are heavily in your favor, are strongly skewed in your behalf, are very much for your achieving total success.

Remember, it's just as anxious a time for your family. They have had to suffer through long hours of waiting and not knowing. All that time you were being prepared for the operation, and then were being taken to the operating room, and perhaps held there to wait until it was your turn, and then, perhaps, the time you spent recovering, before they could see you, was a very anxious, very uncertain time for them. So it is now, they are there to cheer you up and to keep you company, but they will soon lose their cheer if you are glum and pessimistic. Instead, you have to be positive and optimistic for their sake. Of course, your doctor will help. As soon as the operation is completed, he will go out to your family and tell them what he did and what he found and assure them that you are resting and doing well.

When that dramatic time comes to remove the bandages, your heart will be leaping and you may be biting your lip. That is quite natural. Just remember that, even though your opening your eye may not prove as dramatic as it did for Clyde, the Milwaukee man whose case we narrated in the first chapter, your vision will get better in the days and weeks ahead. Also, if you look closely with a mirror at the incisions and stitches you will see puffy, unattractive tissue. Give it a chance. It takes months to heal. Once the healing process is completed, you will find it very difficult, if not impossible, to tell where the incision was.

Just when you'll be able to leave the hospital depends on the kind of surgery you had. Your doctor will give you a special set of instructions for caring for your eye and detail ways in which you may have to modify your behavior. We have already told many of these in the chapters on specific eye conditions earlier in the book. But, to recap, here are the conditions, the length of hospitalization and special instructions your doctor may give.

MUSCLE OPERATIONS: Bandage off in twenty-four hours, home in two days, back to school or work in another two days. Mild activities in about a month. Strenuous or bumpy activities in later months. Eye training may be necessary.

CORNEA OPERATIONS: In the hospital for two or three weeks, with bandages changed every day. Both eyes are kept bandaged to keep them immobile so that sutures won't rub against the lids and cause irritation. Your eyes will be kept bandaged. After about three or four months, you'll return to the hospital to have the sutures painlessly removed. This takes about five minutes, and is usually done in the operating room. Your eyes will be bandaged again, in order to let the epithelial tissues grow into the small holes left behind. Then you'll be sent back home, where after about another month the bandages will be permanently removed. You'll probably need contact lenses to see perfectly, but these won't be fitted for another six months.

GLAUCOMA OPERATIONS. You'll have to stay in bed for two days after your eye is operated on, and remain in the hospital for two more days while the eye heals and the doctor tests the pressure of your eyeball to be sure it is reduced. You can go back to work and resume most activities in about two or three weeks. You'll probably have to come back later to have the other eye operated on.

CATARACT OPERATIONS. If he does both during the same hospitalization, your doctor will probably wait two or three days after operating on the first eye to do the other eye, but he'll want you on your feet twenty-four hours after each eye operation. In all, you can expect to be in the hospital for six to nine days. Some doctors prefer to wait a few months between eye operations, in which case you can figure on repeating a four-day hospital stay. The bandages will be changed daily, but don't expect perfect vision with the removal of the first bandages. The world may look brighter, but you won't see things clearly until you get the special glasses (and later contact lenses, perhaps) as we discussed in Chapter 6. The bandages will be protected by a metal eyeshield for four weeks, after which, during a visit to the doctor, he'll take them off. He'll want you to wear the shield at night and the glasses during the day for another few weeks.

RETINA OPERATIONS. If your detached retina is treated by laser, it may be done on an outpatient basis, which will mean you won't even have to be admitted to the hospital or stay overnight. If it is treated with a buckling operation, you can expect to be hospitalized for about four days. If it is treated by hot or cold "spotwelding," you'll have to lie on your back for about a month. Your condition will dictate the treatment and the length of your hospital stay.

TUMOR OPERATIONS. How long you are hospitalized will depend on the kind of tumor, where it is located, and how extensively the tumor has grown. Some small tumors on eyelids can be treated on an outpatient basis. Others (including eye removal) require up to a week in the hospital.

PLASTIC SURGERY. You'll probably need to be in the hospital only overnight and will be able to go home the evening of your operation. The stitches will come out in four to five days. The healing process is slow and visible, so don't expect final results for about six months (as we explained in Chapter 9).

There are some general rules to follow, no matter what the operation. The most pervasive one is: Take It Easy. Don't engage in any strenuous or hectic activities. Move slowly and deliberately. Don't push, pull, or lift anything heavy. At the same time, try to increase your physical activity, mostly by walking. When you are allowed to read or watch television, do it gradually and in small doses. It's a good idea to have your hair cut short *before* the operation, because hair can be very troublesome *after* the operation. In fact, you may not be allowed to wash your hair for weeks. Also, of interest to women, no cosmetics are allowed for several months.

PAYING FOR YOUR OPERATION

As we said early in the book, you have to be prepared to pay for your operation, which means you'll have to pay the hospital, and the doctor, and perhaps an anesthesiologist. You can figure that a semiprivate room these days will cost you about $100 a day. Add another $50 or so for tests and about $100 for the operating room, anesthesia, and so forth. Blue Cross and other group hospital payment plans should cover most, if not all of the hospital bills. Medicare and Medicaid will also pay for necessary eye operations.

As for the surgeon, his bill is for service rendered, which means that his statement will reflect the amount of time he has spent before, during, and after your operation in caring for you. Fees are generally higher in big cities, and on the West Coast, with the highest in Manhattan, Chicago, and Los Angeles, and the lowest in Denver and the South.

It's a good idea to discuss his fee with your surgeon well before the operation, and what it includes—and doesn't. Too many patients are too shy about such talk. Your doctor is really not embarrassed to talk to you about it, and to arrange the most convenient way for you to pay, even over a long period of time, if necessary.

As we said earlier, your doctor will recommend surgery only when he is convinced that it is unavoidable. Any operation is a serious stress for your body. While modern surgery performs wonders, it still should not be taken lightly. It taxes the body and brings you temporary discomfort. But when it is the only thing to do, it can give you a new way of life and a new, bright, and wonderful way of seeing the world again. After all the trouble and expense, it's worth it. Sight is indeed a precious gift.

Index

131